D0178091

Nadia Sawalha

Greedy Girl's Diet

Nadia Sawalha is one of television's busiest presenters. She first came to fame as Annie Palmer in BBC TV's *EastEnders* in the late 1990s, then switched to TV presenting as one of the original line-up of ITV's award-winning *Loose Women*. Since then, she has presented numerous other shows including *City Hospital, Eating in the Sun, Passport to the Sun* and *Wanted Down Under*.

In 2007, she won *Celebrity MasterChef* and quickly became one of the country's most in-demand foodies. She is author of the best-selling cookbook *Stuffed Vine Leaves Saved My Life* and is currently the food columnist for the *Daily Mirror* and *Best* and *Closer* magazines.

She is a regular presenter on ITV's flagship show *Lorraine* and recently co-presented ITV Breakfast's *Saturday Cookbook*.

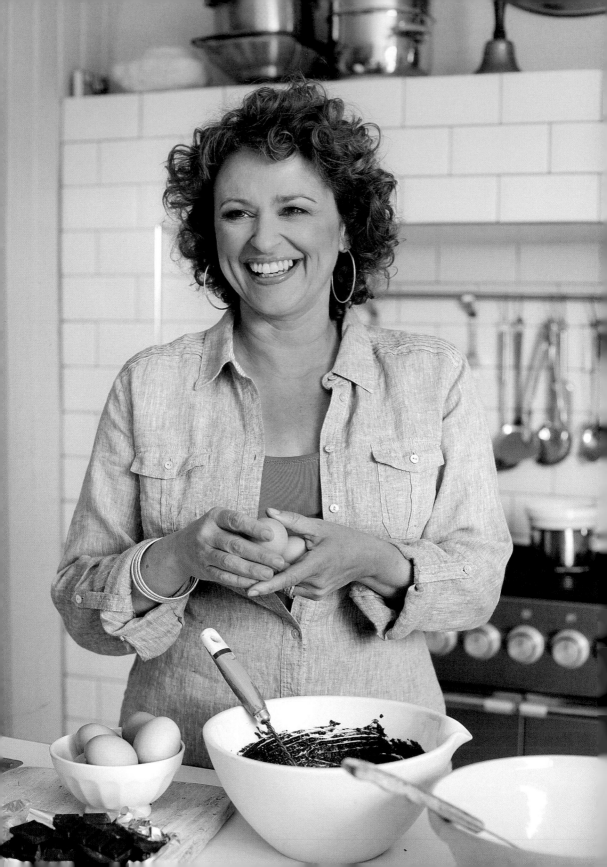

Nadia Sawalha

Greedy Girl's Diet

Eat yourself slim with gorgeous, guilt-free food

Photography by Keiko Oikawa

KYLE BOOKS

For my Mark, whose unfailing belief in me has given me the courage to make all my dreams come true. x

First published in Great Britain in 2013 by
Kyle Books, an imprint of Kyle Cathie Ltd
23 Howland Street
London W1T 4AY
general.enquiries@kylebooks.com
www.kylebooks.com

10 9 8 7 6 5 4 3 2 1

ISBN 978 0 85783 089 0

Text © 2013 Nadia Sawalha
Design © 2013 Kyle Books
Photographs © 2013 Keiko Oikawa

Notes on Nutrition

The nutritional information given with each recipe is given per serving. It does not take into account salt added as in 'salt and pepper' as the amount you add is discretionary. This means that the salt content for each dish is before the seasoning salt it added. Serving suggestions (e.g. 'Low-fat Greek yogurt, to serve') are not included in the analyses.

Nadia Sawalha is hereby identified as the author of this work in accordance with Section 77 of the Copyright, Designs and Patents Act 1988.

All rights reserved. No reproduction, copy or transmission of this publication may be made without written permission. No paragraph of this publication may be reproduced, copied or transmitted save with written permission or in accordance with the provisions of the Copyright Act 1956 (as amended). Any person who does any unauthorised act in relation to this publication may be liable to criminal prosecution and civil claims for damages.

Project Editor: Judith Hannam
Editorial Assistant: Tara O'Sullivan
Copy Editor: Catherine Ward
Designer: Heidi Baker
Photographer: Keiko Oikawa
Cover Photographer: Nicky Johnston
Food Stylist: Polly Webb-Wilson
Prop Stylist: Iris Bromet
Hair and Make Up: Simone Vollmer
Clothes Styling: Fiona Parkhouse
Production: Lisa Pinnell

LANCASHIRE COUNTY LIBRARY	
3011812551694 2	
Askews & Holts	21-Dec-2012
613.25082 SAW	£14.99

A Cataloguing in Publication record for this title is available from the British Library.

Colour reproduction by ALTA London
Printed in Hong Kong by 1010 Printing Group Ltd

Contents

My Secret

By my calculations, I have wasted exactly half my life living in fear. The sad thing is we all know I'm not the only one!

Fear of what?, I hear you ask. Well, fear that I would never reach the 'perfect size 10'. Fear that ultimately, no matter what else I have achieved in my life, I would forever be a complete failure as a woman if I never lost the right amount of weight. This fear has been a cruel master residing in my head for as long as I can remember, and it has always kept me just where it wanted me – directly under its thumb. I would wake up to its nastiness and fall asleep to it still nagging in my ears. It was the fear and self-loathing that kept me overfed physically, but emotionally and spiritually starving. A wise person once said, FEAR stands for False Evidence Appearing Real. How true. False evidence that had quite literally ruled most of my adult life, enslaving my mind and my body. That's no exaggeration. I was a total slave.

I spent years starving, bingeing, starving, bingeing and then starving and bingeing all over again, to no avail. Sound nuts, huh? Well, it is really. To keep repeating the same action whilst expecting a different outcome is quite literally the definition of insanity!

Without realising it, I had thrown away years of my life, believing all the promises the diet industry made: the quick fixes that would make all my dreams come true; the endless new weight-loss 'solutions'; the diets that were rumoured to be 'celebrity' favourites. All of them were right up there at the top of my loons list. You know the ones I mean, the diets that promise that all we have to do is follow them to the letter and we, too, can be as rich, famous, gorgeous or successful as whoever's arse they were claiming to have reduced with this or that particular brand of magic! Most of these diets are now so famous, even my cat could tell you what you can and can't eat on them. The Atkins diet; the boiled egg and grapefruit diet; the Zone diet; the blood group diet; the blah blah blah diet...

After the celebrity diets, my next favourites were the ones that I like to call the 'mock medicals'. The Mayo Clinic diet; the Scarsdale diet; and let's not forget the greatest mock medical of them all, the diet 'rumoured' to have got our very own Princess Catherine 'picture

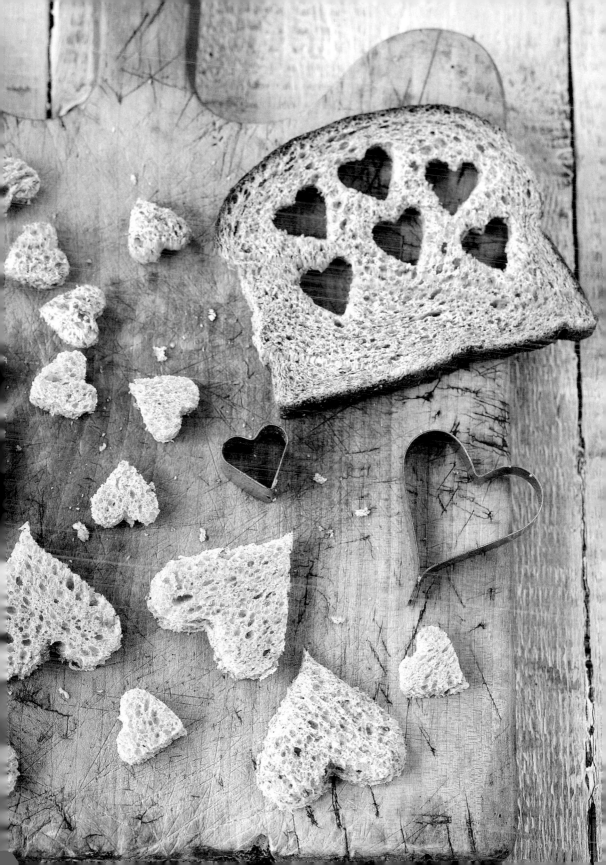

perfect' for Prince William, the Dr Dukan (or the Dr Do-CAN'T as I prefer to call it!) diet. Yep, I've done them all, and guess what... they didn't work. Not one of them.

That's not to say I didn't lose weight on any of them, because I did. But – and it's a big BUT – I always put it all back on, PLUS a bit more! And on top of it all, I felt at least 20 times more miserable after each failed attempt. I felt like I was a hamster (a size 16–18 hamster!) on the never-ending wheel of weight-loss. I was living with the enemy and yet, at the same time, I *was* the flaming enemy.

But, thank God, you'll be pleased to know that this rather miserable sob story does have a happy ending – one in which I discovered a secret that, quite frankly, emancipated me from diet slavery. Yes, that's right. At the age of 45, I had a light bulb moment.

It came out of the blue on an ordinary day. It was a beautiful sunny afternoon and I was chasing my three-year-old

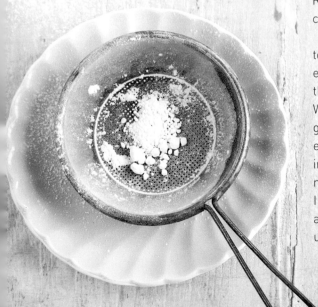

daughter up the stairs. She was giggling in the way three-year-olds do, full of energy and fun, and I was hit by the stark difference between us. Kiki was jumping about with an enviable vitality, whereas I looked like I was going to need a stretcher and some intravenous gin to get back down the stairs! Old at just 45. As I sat there, waiting to recover, I asked myself a serious question. Apart from the age difference, what else was different about Kiki and I that meant she was so full of energy and yet I was practically a goner? Well, pretty quickly I was struck with the obvious answers.

Firstly, she had had a delicious breakfast of homemade buckwheat pancakes, blueberries and thick creamy Greek yogurt. I, on the other hand, had had a mug of tea and half a chocolate digestive. Secondly, she had run around for at least an hour in the garden before eating a gorgeous cottage pie with broccoli and piles of herby carrots for lunch. I, by contrast, had had four Ryvitas, a boiled egg , three pieces of cake and a crafty bag of crisps.

Not for the first time in my life I had to ask myself if I was mad. Why hadn't I eaten the same as her in order to have the energy to run, jump and love life? What made me think that I was ever going to be slim and healthy, while I was eating what I was eating? And, most importantly, why was I able to nourish my daughter's body, but not my own? I realised there and then that I was sick and tired of feeling sick and tired. I faced up to the fact that food, for most of my life, had been more like a drug; a drug with which I punished and rewarded myself, but never nourished myself.

I'd always loved cooking. I come from a family of great cooks. I also (like so many cooks) rather absurdly rarely ate my own food. So, invariably, as my family tucked into an array of gorgeous dishes, I would, more often than not, shun them, nibbling on 'diet food' and having mini-binges as I did the washing-up. Did I really think the calories wouldn't count if nobody saw me devouring them?!

' That's when I decided enough was enough.'

I wasn't going to start a new diet tomorrow. I wasn't going to start a new diet ever again. I decided, then and there, as Kiki bounced before me full of life, that I was going to go back downstairs and cook something simple, delicious and good for me for supper that night. I was going to eat it with my whole family and, most importantly, I was going to continue to do that for the rest of my life. No more quick fixes.

I phoned my friend Julia to ask for her help and the very next day, very, very slowly, I began to run. And I continued to exercise every day. Every day I continued to eat delicious food, telling myself that it was what my body deserved in order to live life to the full. I ate without guilt. I began to nourish my amazing body that

had borne my girls; that had served me; that had waited patiently for me to stop hating it and punishing it and finally start treating it in the manner it deserved! And as soon as I did, my body responded.

That was two years ago, and since then I have lost and kept off three and a half stone, all by simply throwing away the diet books and eating three gorgeous nourishing meals a day, every day; by eating the same food as my family, by never counting calories; by cooking all the dishes my family and I love.

I simply shaved off the hidden calories. A little less oil here, a different cut of meat there, brown rice instead of white, more herbs, spices and colour, and a dessert EVERY day. Yep, you heard me correctly! I steadily and gradually lost the weight. My husband also lost two stone, and we didn't even know he was fat! I am free from the fear and loathing, and I can't believe how easy and obvious the answer was. I simply returned to my family motto of 'good food cooked with love feeds the soul as well as the body', except I would like to change this saying now to 'good food cooked with love for YOURSELF feeds the soul as well as the body'. I am unashamed to admit that I feel truly evangelical about this.

There are over a hundred recipes in this book that will nourish and treat you and your family. Follow my way and you too can have, if not a 'perfect body', certainly a fit and healthy one. Like me, you truly deserve to have and to hold the very same verve and vitality that any three-year-old would take for granted!

Exercise

As I sit down to write about my relationship with (DIRTY WORD ALERT) 'exercise', I feel more than a little nervous.

You see, if I can't inspire you with what I'm about to say, I will have failed you, and betrayed the faith you put in me when you bought this book. As I've already told you, I have read every diet book imaginable since my teens.

I would love nothing more than to settle down on the sofa (often munching on something quite fattening) and lap up the pages of dieting success stories, convinced that somehow their success would magically become my own. I would pore over the recipes, jotting down the lists of dos and don'ts as if my life depended on it. I would memorise the so-called 'forbidden' and 'allowed' foods. But there would always be one chapter in each of these dieting 'bibles' that I would skip, no matter what – and that was the EXERCISE chapter. I would unashamedly flick past it without a second thought. The reason? Arrogance? Denial? Laziness? Fear? Insecurity?

Well, I can honestly say that I used every bloody one of those excuses. I really believed that I, unlike any other person on the planet, could somehow lose weight and get toned up without doing any exercise whatsoever!

Remarkable. And how could I have lived for quite so long with so much denial? Put simply, it was because it suited me. Yes, it suited me to lie down instead of sit down, to walk instead of run and to lounge instead of play. I was lazy, and the reason I was lazy was because I was undernourished. Years of overeating and crash dieting had got my fat arse very firmly stuck in the armchair!

So when the 'lightbulb moment' happened that day on the stairs, I knew everything had to change. I had to change not only the way I ate but also the way I looked after myself. As a result, there was no escaping the fact that, at some point, I was going to HAVE to exercise! Aggh! No! Please, anything but that! The prospect of it (as you've probably gathered) filled me with utter dread. I was terrified at the thought of it. Terrified that all the excuses I had used over the years to keep me from being fit and healthy had to be binned. I could no longer tell myself that exercise was bad for my knees, my heart and my family. There could be no more 'tomorrows' because tomorrow had never come. There was never going to be a perfect day to 'begin' to exercise! Consequently I could have laughed my head off (if I hadn't been crying) when on my very first venture out for a run with my friend Julia, the day could not have been less perfect. It was pouring with rain, I had the hangover from hell and a pair of rotten old plimsoles on, which I had matched with a rotten old tracksuit with no real waist elastic to speak of. I know for certain that if Julia hadn't been waiting for me I would have waddled straight back home for a cup of tea and a biscuit (or ten). But that wasn't an option.

'I had made a promise to myself.'

Well, that first session was not pretty; I could only manage to run for thirty seconds and then I had to walk for three minutes to recover enough to run for another thirty seconds. I felt fat and ugly, but by the end of that forty-five minutes I can honestly say... I still felt fat and ugly... ha ha, got you there! But a seed had been sown, a seed that held a promise that maybe, just maybe, if I came out the next day and the day after that, my life would begin to change.

For weeks, come rain or shine, I would pull on my tracky bottoms and plimmys whilst moaning and groaning and telling myself that, no matter what, I HAD to get out there and exercise. But then one day, out of the blue, the most

bizarre thing happened. I realised that I WANTED to go to my exercise session. In fact, I was looking forward to it!

(DANGER: DO NOT GIVE UP READING THIS SECTION.)

Yep, I was falling in love with exercise. And not just because the fat was melting off my body, but because I felt energised, empowered, ecstatic.

When I look back, I wonder why I was so reluctant to exercise. Why could I not bring myself to step out and get fit? Well, the reason was as old as the hills – an unhealthy diet, too much booze and a ready excuse not to partake in any kind of exercise on offer were clouding my judgement. Dance classes were a no-no because I was convinced that everyone in the class would be looking at me – what an egomaniac! They were there to dance, have fun and get fit, not to look at my miserable mug! Power walking was out, simply because I thought people looked 'silly' when they were power walking! I couldn't choose tennis as an option because, wait for it, I hadn't learnt to play it at school! The point I'm trying to make is that I spent years dreaming up the weirdest and most wonderful excuses I could to get out of exercising when, in fact, all I was getting out of was feeling bloody brilliant! Simple as that. So, stop the excuses! Make a promise today. Make it now. This very minute. Say to yourself, 'exercise is now going to be part of my life for the rest of my life!' – not because it HAS to be, but because you WANT it to be.

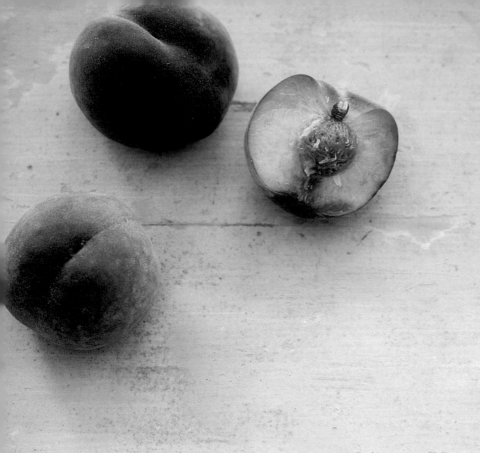

'Breakfast is a great time for any greedy girl to feast without guilt – and we don't want to miss out on an opportunity to do that, do we?'

Come on, Break that Fast

Come on, Break that Fast

Right, let's get started on a brand new road, a wonderful new way of thinking, and what better place to start than by looking at how vitally important a good breakfast is to maintaining a healthy mind and body.

Firstly, breakfast is a great time for any greedy girl to feast without guilt – and we don't want to miss out on an opportunity to do that, do we? After all, you won't have eaten anything for at least eight hours, unless of course you can sleep-eat (mmm... now there's an idea to go alongside sleepwalking). Just imagine a truly greedy girl going without anything to eat for the same amount of time in daylight hours? That would clearly be crazy! And yet, millions of us choose to go without breakfast every day. So come on girls, let's take full advantage of the situation and really investigate all the glorious food we can indulge in to break that dreadful self-imposed fast.

One (and believe me there have been many) of the biggest mistakes I made as a fat greedy girl, rather than a slimmer greedy girl, was that I would routinely skip breakfast, foolishly thinking that it would be the best start to my 'dieting' day! I'm sure many of you will be able to identify with my somewhat warped way of thinking... so, let me hit the play button on the internal voice that is my dieting mind: 'Right, OK, if I miss brekkie that will save me 300 calories, and then if I have a light lunch and a really, really good power walk with just a healthy

dinner I will definitely have lost a few pounds by tomorrow'. What a clever bird I was, eh? I had a plan and it was going to bring me eternal happiness and the body I had always dreamed of (and, who knows, maybe even world peace, too). It never once occurred to me that there was anything remotely silly about this approach, even though this daily deceit had got me absolutely nowhere in my quest to release the beautiful, sexy me that was trapped under layers of fat!

They say that insanity is repeating the same action always expecting a different outcome. I was clearly insane. Day in, day out, I would begin my day truly believing that this was it. Today, I would pull it off and be on the road to Mecca. But day after day, come 10 o'clock, I would find myself ramming something down my throat (always at great speed so that no one, not even myself, could see me) – and that one snack would, of course, amount to infinitely more calories than a delicious, healthy, nourishing breakfast. From here on, the day would ALWAYS go from bad to worse. Hmm... there's that insane feeling again.

Next, lunchtime would arrive – and, with it, the guilt of the earlier feeding frenzy. I would demurely refuse anything to eat, claiming I was watching my weight, to which there would often be looks of bemusement from my colleagues (which, of course, I would read as looks of approval because of that insane voice in my head again!).

Clearly with no nourishment in my system other than a doughnut, the whole idea of the power walk I had so naively planned to do during my lunch break gently faded away.

'A doughnut, although bloody lovely, doesn't give you much energy.'

Anyway, my 'dieting' day would continue to discombobulate itself with endless stolen nibbles and snacks, leaving me fat and overstuffed, but, rather sadly, completely undernourished and consequently utterly exhausted. So... what would I do to remedy this? Why, when I got home I'd open a bottle of wine, of course! Genius! Don't forget, folks, that wine was invented by the Romans to 'open the appetite'. So I would sip my wine while preparing an utterly delicious meal for my family, but because I would still be ravenously hungry, and without any sense of how nuts I was being, I would start slicing off hunks of bread, dipping them into the delicious sauce bubbling on the stove, scoff a lump of cheese, finish off the crisps in the girls'

lunchbox, devour a banana, sneak a piece of dry stale cake, and on and on it would go... until dinner was ready.

Finally, I would sit down with my family – once again overstuffed, undernourished and, if I'm honest, a bit pissed – and announce that I wasn't hungry, and anyway I didn't want to eat because... wait for it... I was on a diet! Brilliant! Genius! How different the day would have been, and could have been, if I'd only just had the willpower to break my fast properly and nourish my body.

This chapter contains a selection of the breakfasts I ate (and will now continue to eat for the rest of my life) when things finally 'clicked' for me. I firmly believe it is impossible to lose weight and keep it off without eating a damn fine breakfast every single day. I also think that variety is the spice of life; it's all too easy to get stuck eating the same thing day in day out. Breakfast should be more fun than that! After all, it's the first time we restart our daily relationship with food. So it should be interesting AND rewarding.

Never leave the table too hungry or too stuffed. It's always a good idea to leave the breakfast table with a piece of fruit and a small handful of seeds in case you get a greedy attack mid-morning. Be prepared, that's my motto!

There is a breakfast here for every occasion, so there's no excuse to skip it. Come on, turn that frown upside down into a smile and feast on a gorgeous breakfast – your mind, body and soul deserve it!

Lazy Weekends

Beautiful Berry Pancakes

Although my husband Mark and I love, occasionally, to tuck into a full Sunday fry-up, our girls most definitely do not! So, as it's Sunday and I'm a top-dollar mama, I make these Beautiful Berry Pancakes for them to tuck into instead! My top tip for topping these is to use agave syrup rather than sugar or golden syrup, as it doesn't cause the dreaded sugar crash that can leave you starving an hour after you've eaten. I must stress that these pancakes are most definitely NOT only for children, BUT stick to just two, or maybe three if you have some exercise planned.

Serves 4 (makes 8 pancakes)

2g FAT | 0.5g SATURATES | 5.7g SUGARS | 0.53g SALT | 153 CALORIES

125g self-raising flour
2 teaspoons caster sugar
½ teaspoon baking powder
small pinch of salt
1 egg, separated
150ml skimmed milk
1 teaspoon vanilla extract
vegetable oil spray
50g blueberries or raspberries

To serve
1 tablespoon icing sugar
agave syrup

Put the flour, caster sugar, baking powder and salt into a mixing bowl. Combine the egg yolk with the milk and vanilla extract in a jug and whisk into the dry ingredients until you have a smooth batter. In a separate bowl, whisk the egg white until soft peaks form and carefully fold into the batter.

Heat a non-stick frying pan and spray with a thin film of oil. Put a spoonful of the pancake mixture into the pan and sprinkle a few blueberries or raspberries on top. Once you see bubbles forming, flip the pancake and cook on the other side. Transfer to a warm plate while you finish cooking the rest. To serve, dust with icing sugar and accompany with agave syrup.

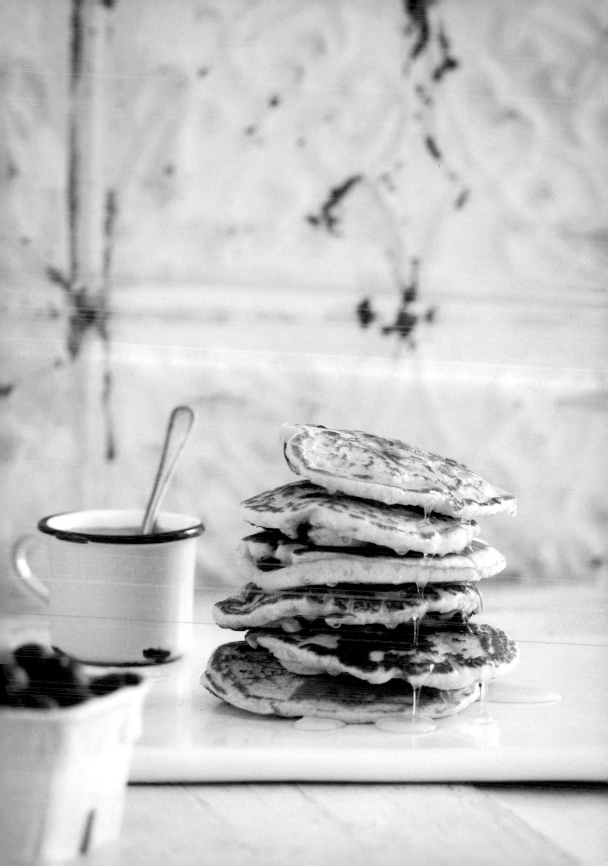

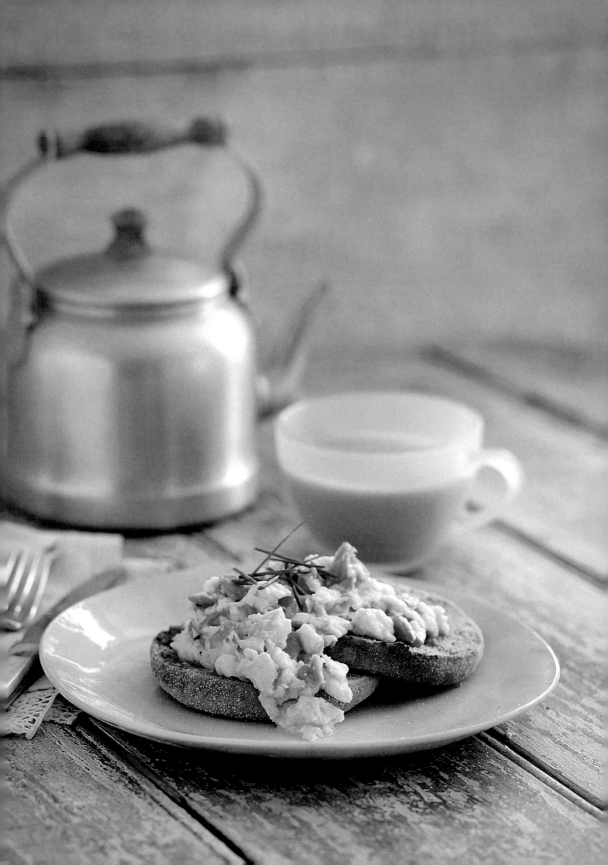

Scrambled Egg and Smoked Trout

I prefer to use smoked trout with scrambled eggs rather than the more traditional smoked salmon because I find it less fatty, but feel free to use either. You can play around with the herbs if you fancy. Maybe some fresh thyme or parsley instead of the chives? Try to buy the best eggs possible. Not only are they better for you, but also they taste better than cheaper varieties.

Serves 4	16g FAT	4.6g SATURATES	0.7g SUGARS	1.94g SALT	310 CALORIES

200g smoked trout or salmon
2 tablespoons reduced-fat cream
8 eggs
black pepper
2 tablespoons chopped chives
2 teaspoons light butter
2 wholemeal muffins

Using a pair of scissors, cut the smoked trout into small pieces and put into a little bowl. Pour the cream over the top. Leave to infuse for 20 minutes to soften the fish and add extra creaminess.

Lightly whisk the eggs and add a little black pepper and the chives, reserving some to sprinkle on the top. Melt the light butter in a non-stick pan, pour in the eggs and keep stirring until they are half-cooked. Add the smoked trout and cream and continue to stir until the eggs are cooked.

Toast the muffins and serve 1 half per person with the scrambled eggs on top. Don't forget to sprinkle the reserved chives on top.

The Great British Fry-Up

I love nothing more on a lazy Sunday morning than a big fry-up; the only thing is I don't actually like it fried any more! I think bacon, sausage and tomato all taste so much better grilled, which is very fortunate because, of course, it's a far healthier way to eat them. I will admit, though, I do sometimes give in to a wee bit of fried bread!

Serves 4	14g FAT	4.1g SATURATES	2.4g SUGARS	2.03g SALT	259 CALORIES

20 cherry tomatoes, on the vine
salt
olive oil spray
3–4 sprigs of fresh thyme (or a
few pinches of dried thyme)
4 lean sausages
4 rashers of lean back bacon
4 eggs
4 slices of wholemeal toast with
a scraping of low-fat spread

Preheat the oven to 220°C/gas mark 7 and preheat the grill to moderate.

Put the tomatoes on a baking tray. Sprinkle with salt and spray with olive oil. Throw in the thyme and roast in the oven for 15–20 minutes. (Alternatively, pop them under the grill with the sausages – see below.)

Place the sausages on a grill tray and set under the grill for 15–20 minutes until browned and cooked through, turning once. After 10–15 minutes, add the bacon – and, if you're grilling them, the tomatoes. It should take 5–6 minutes for the bacon to cook through and start to go crispy. Turn the tomatoes when they begin to brown on one side.

Meanwhile, poach the eggs. Bring a small pan of water to a gentle rolling simmer, carefully crack in the eggs and cook for about 3 minutes. Drain and serve on top of the toast. Drain the sausages and bacon on kitchen paper and divide between the plates. Serve the tomatoes on the side.

Creamy Scrambled Eggs

Sometimes, only the comfort of deliciously creamy scrambled eggs will do.

| Serves 4 | 13g FAT | 3.6g SATURATES | 3.4g SUGARS | 0.84g SALT | 236 CALORIES |

4 medium tomatoes, halved
8 eggs
1 tablespoon skimmed milk
2 teaspoons light butter
2 dessertspoons Philadelphia
  Extra Light cream cheese
4 slices of rye, wholemeal or
  granary bread

Preheat the grill to moderate and grill the tomatoes for 5–7 minutes, turning once, until soft.

Meanwhile, make the scrambled eggs. Beat the eggs and milk together in a bowl. Melt the butter in a non-stick pan, pour in the egg mixture and cook until the eggs are softly set, stirring constantly. Remove from the heat and stir in the cream cheese. Toast the bread, spoon the scrambled eggs on top and serve with those delicious grilled tomatoes on the side.

VARIATION: First spread the toast with a teaspoon of peanut or almond butter. Alternatively, mash up ½ avocado with 1 tablespoon Marmite to make 'marmacado' spread. Spread on the toast and top with the scrambled eggs.

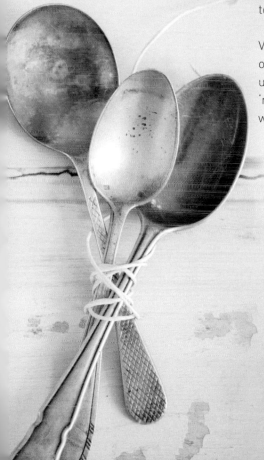

Herby Tomato and Ham Omelette

My dad used to make this delicious omelette for my sisters and me when we were kids, except he used to add garlic to it, too! It was a miracle we had any friends, the way we used to pong! I have kindly omitted the garlic from the ingredients, but feel free to add some if you wish.

Serves 4	12g FAT	3.3g SATURATES	0.2g SUGARS	1.06g SALT	178 CALORIES

8 eggs

4 teaspoons chopped fresh herbs (or use 2 teaspoons dried herbs) – you can use any herbs you like such as parsley, basil, chives or coriander

4 slices of ham with all visible fat removed, chopped

pinch of salt and pepper

olive oil spray

To serve

4 slices of granary bread, toasted

4 tomatoes, sliced

Whisk the eggs and herbs together in a mixing bowl, add the ham and season with a pinch of salt and pepper.

Spray a non-stick pan with a fine mist of oil. Pour in the egg mixture and cook gently for 3–4 minutes, tipping the pan from side to side to allow the uncooked egg to run over the edges of the cooked egg and cook through. Serve with the toast and some sliced tomatoes on the side.

'Buy the best quality ingredients you can afford and sit down and relish every mouthful.'

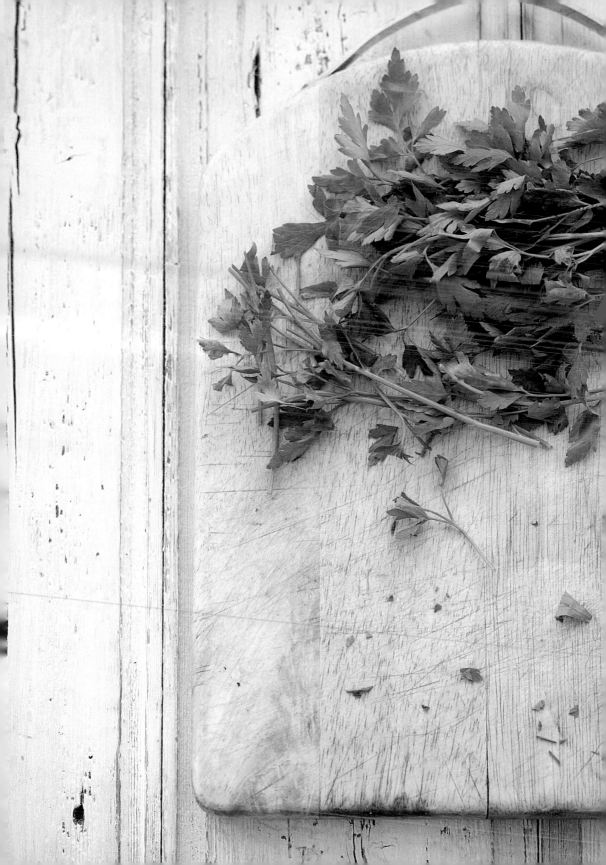

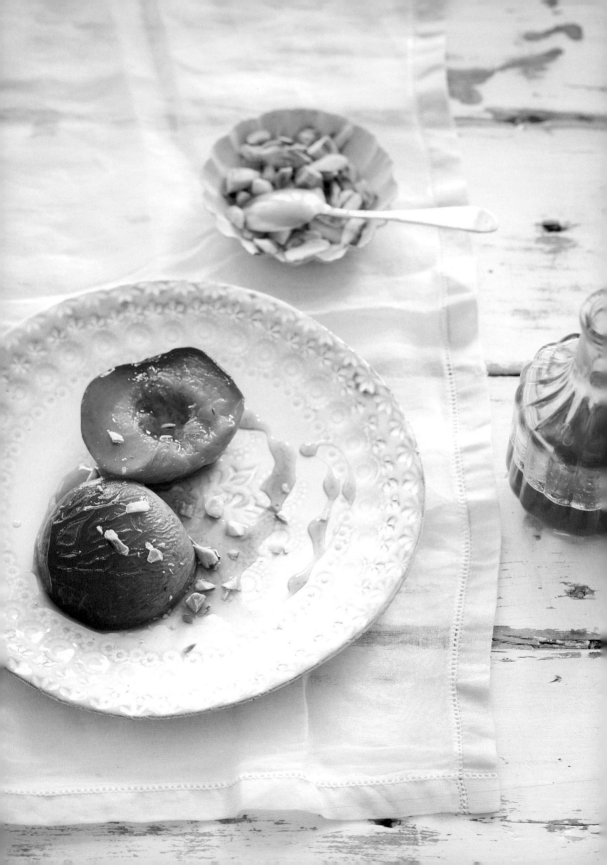

Baked Peaches with Honey, Roasted Almonds and Orange Flower Water

I am a shameless show off, so this is my 'go-to' summer recipe if I have friends staying over, as it never fails to impress people with its beauty. It not only looks beautiful with the peaches glistening in honey topped with golden roasted almonds, but the orange flower water gives it a gorgeously exotic taste and aroma that has people oohing and ahhing. I expect nothing less than a round of applause for this dish!

Serves 4	6g FAT	0.5g SATURATES	16.4g SUGARS	0.01g SALT	129 CALORIES

4 ripe peaches, peeled, halved and stoned

2 tablespoons orange blossom honey

4 tablespoons orange flower water

4 tablespoons chopped roasted almonds

To serve
low-fat Greek yogurt (optional)

Preheat the oven to 180°C/gas mark 4.

Cut the peaches in half and remove the stones. Place the peaches face-up in a roasting tin, drizzle with the honey and bake for 15–20 minutes until the peaches are tender. Remove from the oven, arrange the peach halves on a serving plate and pour the honey juices from the roasting tin into a small pan. Add the orange flower water, bring to the boil and simmer for a couple of minutes. Pour the mixture over the peaches and top with the roasted almonds. Serve with low-fat Greek yogurt.

Breakfast on the Run

The alarm hasn't gone off (or was slammed off and hurled out the window); the kids are refusing to get up, and when they do they can only find their wellington boots, one sock and half a school tie (don't ask!); the guinea pigs, cat, kids and husband all want breakfast, packed lunches and clean socks; AND you haven't done your make-up; PLUS you were supposed to have left for work 10 minutes ago. Are you going to ensure you have a delicious, nourishing breakfast that will give you the power to deal with the day? I suspect not. Am I right? Well, never fear, Nads is here with the perfect solution to your misery!

Fabulously Fruity Fun Smoothie

Serves 4 | 1g FAT | 0.2g SATURATES | 26.7g SUGARS | 0.18g SALT | 132 CALORIES

This smoothie will take no more than three or four minutes to whizz up and if you grab a handful of nuts to munch on at the same time you will have an even more filling, nutritious and, quite frankly, angelic breakfast.

4 small pears, cored and
    chopped
4 peaches, halved and stoned
4 apricots, halved and stoned
1 banana
600ml skimmed or soya milk

Place all the ingredients in a blender and whizz together to give a delicious smoothie consistency. Serve in chilled glasses.

Breakfast Literally On the Run

1 avocado
1 bottle of water

Peel and eat while running for the bus, down the bottle of water and you are set up until lunch!

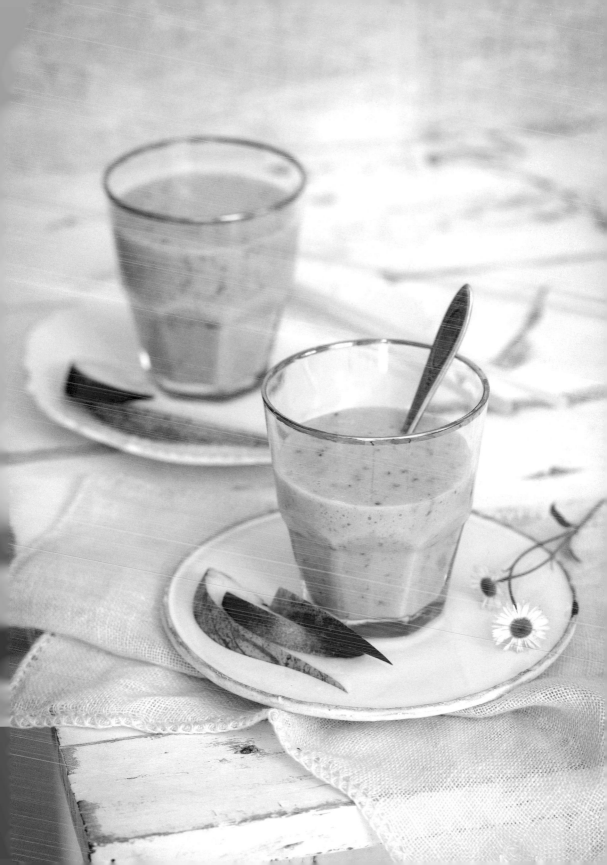

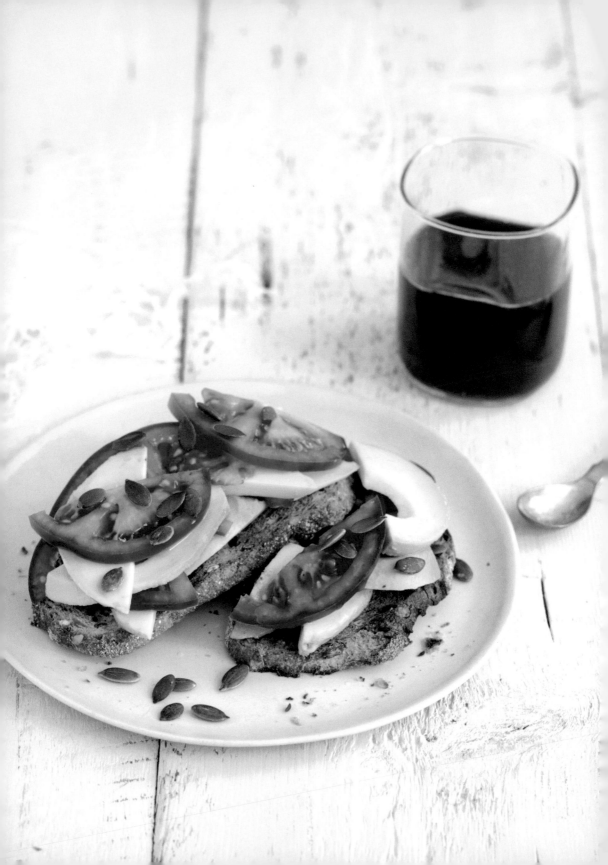

Goody Two-Shoes Vegetable Juice with Nutty Avocado Toast

Don't fear vegetable juice. It really tastes a lot better than you would think and if you have it first thing it leaves you feeling clean and virtuous all day – which means you are far less likely to want to eat anything that's bad for you! Whenever I have a glass of this wonderjuice I show off about it all day to whomever I meet. I get such a kick out of the way people react when I tell them I've made my own vegetable juice and had it for breakfast, it's like they suddenly see me as a beacon of veggie virtue!

Serves 4	14g FAT	3g SATURATES	9.7g SUGARS	0.79g SALT	285 CALORIES

For the vegetable juice
1 cucumber, roughly chopped
5 celery sticks, roughly chopped
1 medium beetroot, peeled and
   roughly chopped
1 medium apple, cored and
   quartered (my kids like it with
   apple, but it's optional)
600g spinach or curly kale

For the avocado toast
4 slices of granary bread,
   toasted
1 avocado, sliced
4 medium tomatoes, sliced
4 tablespoons pumpkin seeds

To make the juice, place all the ingredients in a blender and blitz to a smooth purée. Divide between 4 glasses, which will give approx. 200ml per person

To make the avocado toast, top each piece of toast with slices of avocado and tomato and sprinkle with the pumpkin seeds. Serve with the vegetable juice.

Cinnamon Chocolate Banana Shake

Oooh, this is the perfect solution for a greedy girl on the run! It feels so naughty first thing in the morning with the creaminess of the milk and banana and the spiciness of cinnamon, finished off with a luxurious flourish of chocolate. The added bonus is that the whole family loves this little indulgence, so by making this shake you can shut everyone up very quickly!

Serves 4 | 5g FAT | 2.9g SATURATES | 43.7g SUGARS | 0.12g SALT | 247 CALORIES

4 ripe bananas
400ml semi-skimmed milk
1 teaspoon ground cinnamon
1 tablespoon best-quality cocoa powder (70 per cent cocoa solids)
4 tablespoons agave syrup
4 tablespoons grated dark chocolate

Put the bananas, milk, cinnamon, cocoa powder and agave syrup into a blender and blitz until smooth. Pour into glasses and finish with a sprinkling of grated chocolate.

'Decide the night before what you are going to have for breakfast the next day. It feels great to get up with a plan already in place. As someone famous once said: if you fail to plan, then you plan to fail!'

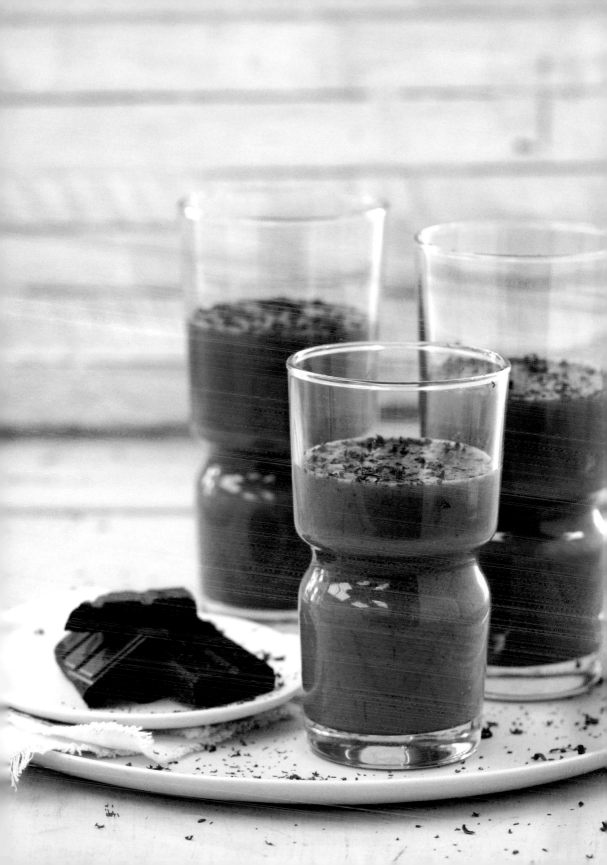

Dr Christy's Power Juice

Now this amazing juice was invented by my very clever friend Dr Christy Fergusson and, believe me, she is so flaming gorgeous she's a brilliant advert for it! This wonderjuice takes just two minutes to make – come on, we can all find two minutes – and I swear every time I have it I can't quite believe a halo doesn't instantly pop up over my head, it's that blooming good for me! Some of the ingredients may make you wonder at my sanity, but please just try it once and feel the power – you will love me for it... or rather, you will love Dr Christy.

Serves 2	14g FAT	2.9g SATURATES	27.4g SUGARS	0.14g SALT	251 CALORIES

1 mango, peeled and stoned

1 cucumber, chopped

50g spinach

1 avocado, peeled and stoned

110–220ml apple juice or
   coconut water

Put the mango, cucumber, spinach and avocado into a high powered blender. Whizz, then add the coconut water or apple juice to thin the mixture to a drinkable consistency.

Jane Wake's Wide Awake Seed Bar

My lovely friend and Pilates trainer Jane Wake created these nifty seed bars because, as a working mother herself, she knows how hard it is to find the time to make a healthy breakfast. And, as a personal trainer, she also knows that it is almost impossible to work out properly on an empty stomach. This little bar of power sorts out the problem.

When I have a spare 15 minutes I make up a batch of them and keep them stored in the back of the larder – hidden rather than stored actually, or Mark (my hubby) would end up munching the lot! The nuts and seeds in them are so good for you, as well as being utterly delicious. I sometimes have a bar as a late-night snack or as a post-workout treat or (because I'm such a greedy guts), sometimes just 'cos I want one!

Makes 12 bars	12g FAT	3.9g SATURATES	11g SUGARS	0.08g SALT	198 CALORIES

50g light butter
140g oats
3 tablespoons honey
50g chopped almonds
50g chopped Brazil nuts
1 tablespoon sunflower seeds
1 tablespoon pumpkin seeds
1 tablespoon sesame seeds
50g finely chopped apricots
50g finely chopped dates
50g desiccated coconut
2 small very ripe bananas,
   mashed

Preheat the oven to 160°C/gas mark 3.

Lightly grease a 22cm square baking tin. Melt the butter, put it in a bowl along with all the other ingredients, and mix well. Pour the mixture into the tin and bake for 30–40 minutes. Leave to cool in the tin for 5 minutes, then cut into 12 bars.

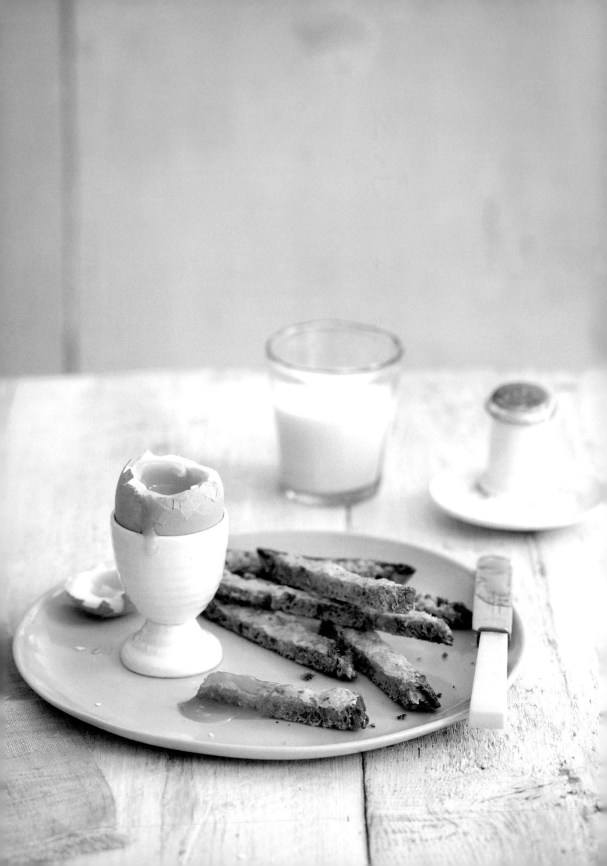

Wake Up to How Wonderful Breakfast Is!

Boiled Eggs with Cheesy Soldiers

Just imagine... gloopy, perfectly boiled eggs with gorgeous cheesy soldiers for dream dippage! This is one of my favourite breakfasts. If I'm really hungry, I have two eggs and that keeps me happy until lunch. I love lunch!

Serves 4	14g FAT	4.3g SATURATES	2.1g SUGARS	0.9g SALT	300 CALORIES

4 free-range eggs
8 slices of wholemeal or
    granary bread
light butter, for spreading
a sprinkling of freshly grated
    Parmesan cheese

Preheat the grill to moderate.

To soft-boil the eggs, place them in a pan and cover with cold water. Bring to the boil over a high heat and, as soon the water reaches boiling point, reduce to a simmer and start your timer – from this point the eggs will take 3–4 minutes to cook, depending on how soft you like them.

Toast 1 side of the bread under the grill, spread the uncooked side with a scraping of butter (heh, a scrape!), sprinkle with the cheese and set under the grill until the cheese melts. Serve each egg with 2 slices of cheesy bread, sliced into soldiers for dipping.

VARIATION: I also like to serve my boiled egg with twiglets (you could also use pretzels) for a twist on egg and soldiers – I call it egg and twigs!

Almond Butter Crumpets

Sometimes, I just want something that feels really junky in the morning and this breakfast, inspired by the famous American peanut butter and jelly sandwich, is the perfect answer. I use almond butter instead of peanut butter because it is much better for you, and reduced-sugar jam to take out some of the naughtiness.

Serves 4   6g FAT | 1.2g SATURATES | 2.1g SUGARS | 1.88g SALT | 239 CALORIES

8 crumpets
8 teaspoons almond butter
8 teaspoons reduced-sugar jam

Simply toast the crumpets and spread each one with a teaspoon of almond butter. Smear each with a teaspoon of jam for an extra junk fix!

Buckwheat Pancakes

These are what I call my 'hardcore' pancakes – they're what I eat when I have a busy day physically, whether that be running around with the kids or at work, or, indeed, going for a long training run. My advice is, don't give these to the kids, because they'll probably throw them at you!

Serves 4	3g FAT	0.6g SATURATES	3.1g SUGARS	0.12g SALT	150 CALORIES

275ml skimmed milk
1 egg
a pinch of salt
1 teaspoon vegetable oil
110g buckwheat flour
vegetable oil spray

To serve
agave syrup
fresh berries

Put the milk, egg, salt and oil into a jug and whisk well. Put the buckwheat flour into a bowl, make a well in the centre and gradually pour in the wet ingredients. Whisk well. Leave to rest in the fridge for half an hour.

Spray a thin mist of oil into a non-stick pan and pour in a small ladleful of the batter. Cook for 1–2 minutes on each side. Repeat until you have used up all the batter (this recipe yields approximately 8 pancakes). Serve topped with a thin drizzle of agave syrup and whatever berries tickle your fancy.

Marathon Muesli

I don't really like most shop-bought mueslis because they often have a lot of added sugar or too much dried fruit. Don't get me wrong – I know they taste nice enough – but after eating a bowlful, your blood sugar can go nuts leaving you with massive cravings. So I like to make my own using plenty of nuts and seeds (as well as a little dried fruit) in addition to energy-giving oats. Mark is a marathon runner and he says a big bowl of this will always get him through the 26.2 miles, so just imagine what it could do for your day!

| Serves 4 | 11g FAT | 4.2g SATURATES | 18.5g SUGARS | 0.14g SALT | 359 CALORIES |

200g porridge oats
1 tablespoon pumpkin seeds
1 tablespoon sunflower seeds
1 tablespoon sesame seeds
8 stoned dates, finely chopped
4 dried apricots, finely chopped
2 tablespoons desiccated coconut
400ml skimmed milk or soya milk (100ml per bowl)
4 tablespoons ground flax seed (optional)

Simply mix together the oats, seeds, dates, apricots and coconut and divide between 4 serving bowls. Pour over the milk and sprinkle with the ground flax seed (if using).

VARIATION: If you prefer, you could swap the milk for 150ml apple juice. Set aside for 5–10 minutes to allow the oats to soak up the juice and soften before eating.

'Empower yourself! Try to think of reasons other than your appearance for eating well – like the importance of feeling fit, energised and empowered.'

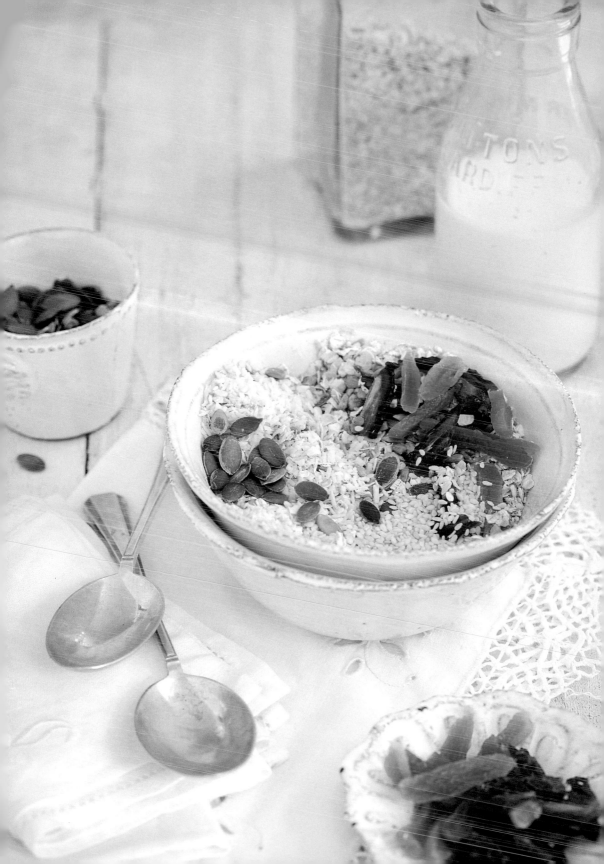

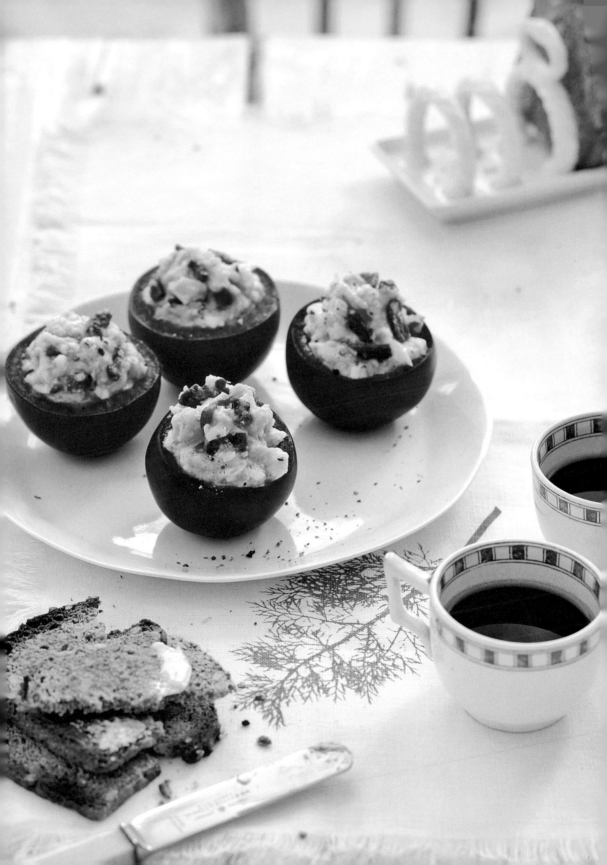

Scrambled Egg and Bacon Tomato Pots

My kids named this dish MY tomato pots; they love the fact they each get their own one. But they're not just for kids – grown ups love them just as much!

Serves 4 | 17g FAT | 4.6g SATURATES | 3.8g SUGARS | 1.41g SALT | 302 CALORIES

4 medium tomatoes

salt

a small knob of light butter

4 rashers of back bacon with all visible fat removed

8 small eggs

a splash of milk

4 slices of wholemeal toast spread with a scraping of light butter

Slice the tops off the tomatoes and spoon out the centres. Sprinkle the insides with a little salt and pop onto 4 plates.

Heat the butter in a non-stick pan, snip the bacon into little pieces and fry for a couple of minutes until crisp, stirring frequently. Meanwhile, lightly whisk the eggs with the milk in a bowl. Pour the egg mixture into the pan with the bacon and stir until the eggs are scrambled the way you like them. Divide the yummy egg mixture between the 4 tomatoes, spooning it into the hollowed-out centres, and serve with hot toast on the side.

A Summer Breeze

Sweet, crisp, ruby red watermelon, fragrant mint leaves and grilled halloumi cheese served with sesame seed bread. Mmm, yes please...

Serves 4	9g FAT	4.7g SATURATES	17.3g SUGARS	2.66g SALT	300 CALORIES

4 thick slices of light halloumi cheese

4 large slices watermelon

a handful of fresh mint

4 slices of sesame seed bread or seeded bread

Heat a griddle pan and cook the halloumi cheese for a couple of minutes on each side until soft. Take 4 plates, and place one slice of watermelon on each. Tear the cheese into strips and scatter over the watermelon. Garnish with a few mint leaves and serve with the sesame seed bread on the side.

'And now for the good news — try to eat something every 3–4 hours. This helps to stabilise your blood sugar and stave off cravings. Take a piece of fruit and a small handful of seeds to work with you every day in case you get a greedy attack mid-morning.'

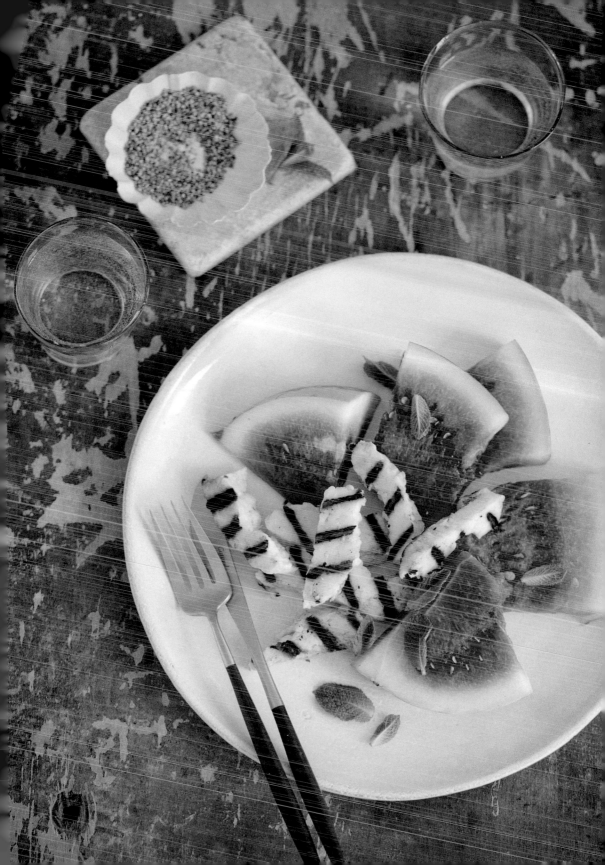

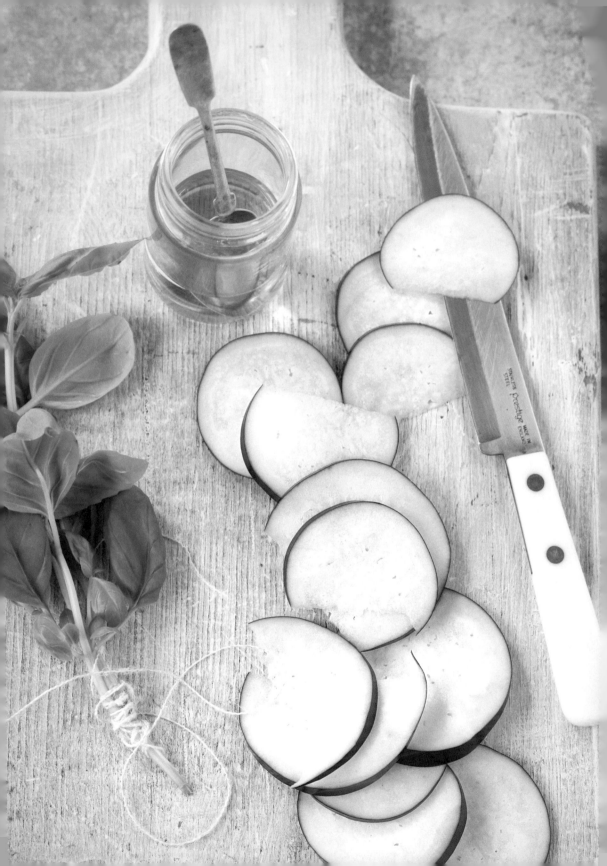

Let's do Lunch

'I want, deserve and need something delicious and nutritious every single day of my life. Firstly, because I love my food and, secondly, because I love being slim!'

Let's do Lunch

Over the 30-year period that I was piling on the pounds the meal I neglected most after breakfast was lunch. When I look back I can mark the decades of my life by the mistakes I made with my diet; mistakes that ensured I steadily and rather impressively gained weight, year after year!

My bad habits well and truly kicked off as a teenager, when I became convinced that I was fat and ugly and the only way that this was ever going to change was if I could successfully diet. I feel such a twit when I look back at photos of myself and see that I was no such thing. In fact, I was quite a babe. What a shame I saw myself more as Babe the pig (from the movie) rather than a babe babe!

In my late teens I was a struggling actress who loved to party and was therefore often still suffering from a hangover at lunchtime. This frequently meant I missed breakfast but, as far as I was concerned, this wasn't really a problem because my twisted way of thinking told me that a missed breakfast was definitely going to mean I'd be thinner by the end of the day. Hooray!

Of course, as I nursed my hangover and felt clever about skipping brekkie, I would have wiped from my mind the memory of the greasy doner kebab I'd devoured at the bus stop the night before – and the fact that I'd poured large amounts of empty calories down my throat with all the booze I'd consumed. Classy, huh?

So, consequently, lunch would often be something I felt I 'deserved' – not only for the 'missed' meal of breakfast but also to help relieve the pain of said hangover. Lunch would therefore entail anything from a sausage sandwich to an utterly disgusting burger. You see, my friends and I had rather cleverly convinced ourselves that there were magical healing properties in a bacon double cheeseburger with sauce (the sauce bit was very important) and, as for a sausage sandwich, well, that was practically a superfood! Denial is a powerful thing, especially if you want to get really, really fat. And, at 17, I was positively gifted in the art of denial.

This 'gift' stayed with me into my twenties and, in fact, when I look back over my twenties I can define them as my craziest dieting years; an entire decade of starving and bingeing. One week I would be on near starvation rations, sticking religiously to some hair-brained diet, and the next I would be stuffing my face, basically due to the fact that, surprise, surprise, I was starving because I had been on a hair-brained diet. Duh!

On a typical dieting day, lunch would consist of anything from half a boiled egg and a handful of watercress to the heady heights of a bowl of cabbage soup.

On a stuffing day, I would go to town with as much high-fat and -sugar food as I could consume. Lunch could be a double cheese and bacon sandwich (white bread, of course) with a big bag of crisps, a large chocolate bar and a hunk of cake! And, of course, a stuffing day would always have to be followed by a starving day, to keep up the insanity.

I remember regularly missing lunch out altogether and really getting off on the 'high' that this feeling of starvation would bring. I felt like I was the coolest chick out there, I was in control, I was a high-flying successful bird that could conquer the world: 'I am thin', I'd shout proudly in my head! Until I heard the screech of tyres braking and had a massive reality check... 'Nope, sorry Nadia – you're deluded! You're not thin at all!' Of course I wasn't, and the reason I wasn't was because of the bloody binges, binges that would always come after a couple of missed meals because, what a surprise (!), I was STARVING.

The ability to manage my weight in my thirties became even harder. We can all 'drop half a stone' fairly easily in our twenties but, my God, that changes in our thirties. My metabolism just seemed to nod off a bit and this is the time I really began to bed down and nurture some good solid fat! The starvation diets became less and less effective and I was starting to panic. To the outside world I was happy (jolly even – you know the stereotype, jolly and fat) and reasonably successful, but behind closed doors I hated myself for still being on the dieting merry-go-round with no flaming idea of how to get off. I was still skipping breakfast and messing up lunch, but I was oblivious to the fact that all I needed to do to be slim, well-nourished and sane was to eat three decent meals and two snacks a day. Not rocket science, I know, but it might as well have been!

In my late thirties I met and married my lovely fella Mark and very quickly (and I mean very quickly) had my daughter Maddie. Now, don't get me wrong, I was making beautiful meals for my family – but being a wife and mother opened up a whole new set of possibilities for messing up my own eating. The pressures of having a new baby and a full-time job meant that I neglected what I was eating for lunch. I simply couldn't see the point of cooking something delicious and nutritious 'just for me', so I would often end up just having a packet of biscuits with big mugs of sweet tea. Breastfeeding had rendered me so knackered that it was just easier to opt for a sugar rush to power me on!

Well, I am very happy to say that since my 'lightbulb moment' (page 8), I am fiercely protective of my lunch. I want, deserve and need something delicious and nutritious every single day of my life. Firstly, because I love my food and, secondly, because I love being slim! Excuse me, I don't know about you, but all this soul searching means I'm just about ready to order lunch now.

Soup, Glorious Soup

Soup is the ultimate guilt-free comfort food. However, I can't stand shop-bought soup – it's often hideously overpriced, highly processed and packed with salt. Homemade soup is one of the easiest things to make, so if you've never tried it before, have a go; you won't look back.

Feel free with all these recipes to chop and change the herbs, spices or vegetables to suit your taste, but what I will say is the secret to a good soup is fresh ingredients, great seasoning and to always fry your base ingredients in a little fat. Simply throwing everything into a pan with a stock cube (as many diet books will tell you to do) will result in 'school-dinner' soup... blergh! Soups are a great on-the-run food. If you're working away from home, you can just put some in a thermos flask and eat it at your desk, or if you're at home for the day you can heat it up and have a nourishing lunch and, more importantly, a really filling meal in minutes. On really hungry days I might have several bowls of soup at lunchtime to prevent any sudden stuffing of those things I may regret!

Creamy Avocado Soup

This soup is so easy to make and absolutely delicious. Now, lots of people on diets fear the great avocado but, I beg you, don't dismiss it from your diet. Although it does contain fat, it's the healthy mono-unsaturated kind. This gorgeous summery chilled soup is packed with calcium and good fats. You can, if you prefer, use it as a dip.

Serves 4	16g FAT	4.4g SATURATES	5.7g SUGARS	0.24g SALT	217 CALORIES

2 ripe avocados, peeled and
    stoned
½ organic cucumber
500g low-fat Greek yogurt
3 tablespoons chopped fresh
    mint, plus extra to garnish

Pop all the ingredients in a blender and blitz until smooth. Transfer the mixture to the fridge for a couple of hours to allow the flavours to really infuse. Serve in a chilled bowl, garnished with extra mint leaves.

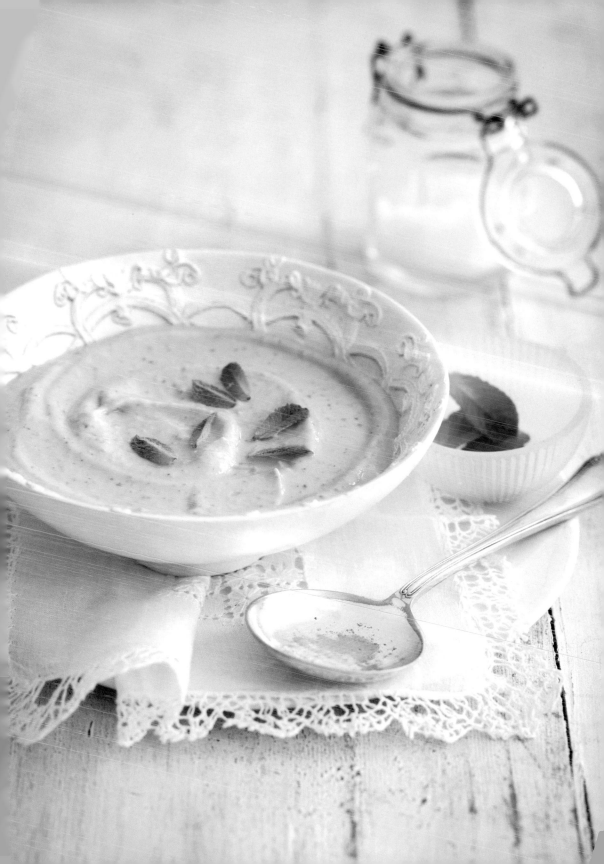

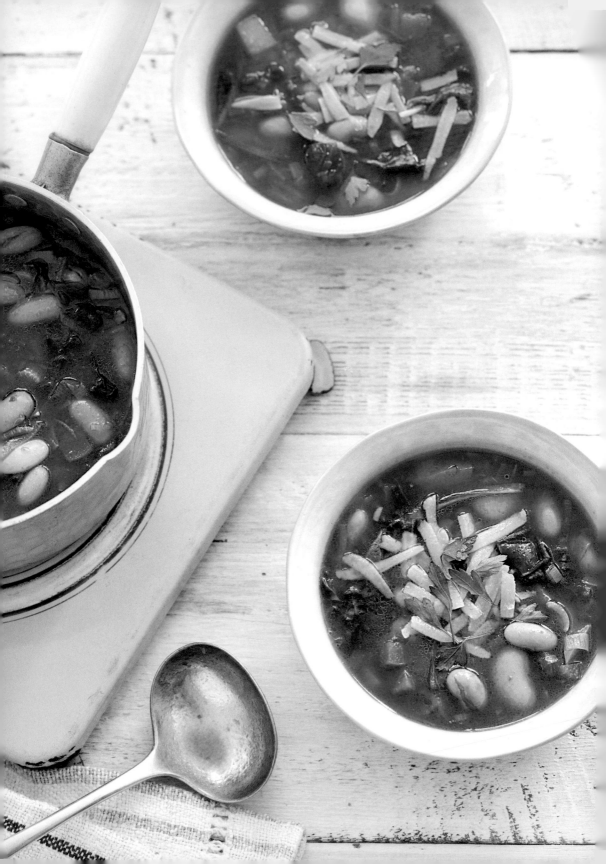

Italian Soup

This soup is very similar to minestrone but, instead of using pasta, I use beans because they're a great source of protein and simply make a nice change from pasta. You could use curly kale instead of spinach if you fancy, which is good if you're a vegan because kale is packed full of calcium. Try to sing a little opera as you serve this to your family. It puts everyone in a great mood... unless you can't sing, of course!

Serves 4	7g FAT	0.9g SATURATES	10.1g SUGARS	0.71g SALT	225 CALORIES

2 tablespoons olive oil

1 large onion, peeled and
    finely chopped

2 celery sticks, finely chopped

2 garlic cloves, peeled and
    finely chopped

3 sprigs of fresh oregano (or
    1 teaspoon dried oregano)

2 carrots, finely chopped

1 leek, trimmed and
    finely chopped

2 medium potatoes, peeled and
    cut into small dice

1 x 400g can white beans (use
    your favourite kind)

250ml chicken or vegetable
    stock

1 x 400g can chopped tomatoes

2 tablespoons finely chopped
    fresh flat-leaf parsley

a large handful of spinach

To serve
freshly grated Parmesan cheese

Heat the oil in a large heavy-based pan, throw in the onion and celery and cook until soft but not coloured. Add the garlic and cook for about 30 seconds, stirring, then throw in the oregano, carrot, leek and potato. Cover and cook over a very low heat for 15 minutes, stirring occasionally.

Once the vegetables are nice and soft, add the beans, stock and tomatoes and simmer really gently for an hour.

Just before you are about to serve, stir in the parsley and spinach leaves and let them wilt. Ladle the soup into bowls and grate over the Parmesan.

Jerusalem Artichoke and Mushroom Soup

This is my mum's recipe and I have to say that when she first told me about it I didn't fancy the sound of it at all – but it's actually really delicious, and the added artichokes make a nice change from a mere mushroom soup.

Serves 4	5g FAT	1.7g SATURATES	8.7g SUGARS	0.8g SALT	208 CALORIES

25g light butter

1 onion, peeled and finely chopped

salt and freshly ground black pepper

1 garlic clove, peeled and crushed or finely chopped

500g Jerusalem artichokes, scrubbed and sliced

1 teaspoon Marigold Bouillon powder dissolved in 400ml hot water

400ml semi-skimmed milk

25g cornflour

250g chestnut mushrooms, cut into small pieces

olive oil spray

1 tablespoon finely chopped fresh flat-leaf parsley

Melt the butter in a large heavy-based saucepan and cook the onion with a pinch of salt until softened but not coloured. Add the garlic and artichokes and fry for a further few minutes. Add the vegetable stock and milk, cover the saucepan with a lid and simmer gently for 25 minutes or until the Jerusalem artichoke pieces are tender. Whizz in a blender until smooth, then return to the pan.

In a small bowl, blend the cornflour with 2 tablespoons cold water. Stir in a few spoonfuls of the soup, then add this mixture to the saucepan. Bring the soup to the boil, stirring continuously until it thickens. Remove from the heat and season to taste.

Heat a little olive oil spray in a frying pan over a medium-high heat and fry the mushrooms until just starting to brown; stir into the soup. Serve in bowls, garnished with chopped parsley.

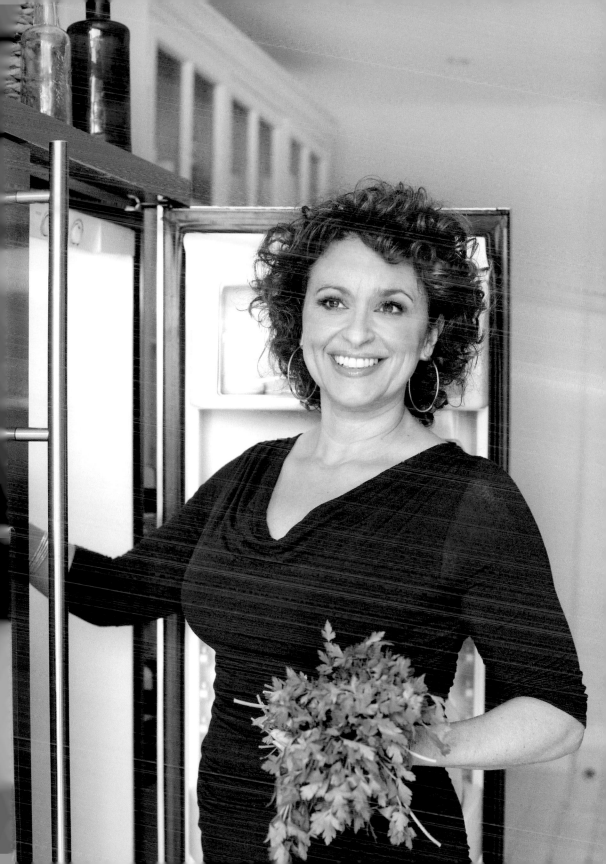

Leek and Potato Soup

I love leek and potato soup! It reminds me of when I was a kid and my mum would make it for us on a Saturday afternoon. We'd come in from playing in the park, freezing cold and happy that mum had stayed at home cooking, because nothing warmed us up in quite the same way as a big bowl of her soup!

Serves 4   4g FAT | 0.7g SATURATES | 5.2g SUGARS | 0.9g SALT | 152 CALORIES

1 tablespoon olive oil
2 rashers of smoked back bacon with all visible fat removed, chopped
1 medium onion, peeled and finely chopped
2 large leeks, trimmed and finely sliced
225g potatoes, peeled and chopped
1 litre chicken stock
salt and freshly ground black pepper
100ml skimmed milk
2 tablespoons chopped fresh chives, to garnish

Heat the oil in a large heavy-based pan and gently fry the bacon, onion and leek until soft. Add the potatoes and stock, bring up to the boil and season with salt and pepper. Cover with a lid and simmer gently until the potatoes are just tender.

Pour the soup into a blender and blitz until you have a lovely smooth soup. Stir in the milk and garnish with chopped chives.

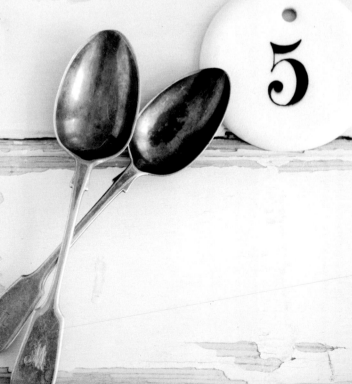

Lentil and Chard Chowder

This recipe makes for a wonderfully soothing supper. If you want to make it more substantial, you could stir in a cup of cooked brown rice or quinoa at the end. You can, of course, also add some cooked chicken if you wish.

Serves 4	4g FAT	0.4g SATURATES	2.5g SUGARS	1.97g SALT	260 CALORIES

150g green lentils, washed
and drained

500ml water

1 teaspoon salt

1 teaspoon ground cumin

500g chard, trimmed and
roughly chopped

3 medium potatoes, peeled
and diced

1 tablespoon olive oil

2 tablespoons finely chopped
onions

1–2 garlic cloves, peeled and
crushed

3 tablespoons finely chopped
fresh coriander

2 teaspoons lemon juice

Put the lentils into a saucepan with the water, salt and cumin, bring to the boil, reduce the heat and simmer for 25 minutes. Add the chopped chard and potato and simmer until tender.

Meanwhile, in a small frying pan, fry the onion in olive oil very slowly until it begins to soften but not colour. Add the garlic and coriander and fry for a further minute. Add this mixture to the lentils, stir in the lemon juice and cook for a further 10 minutes before serving.

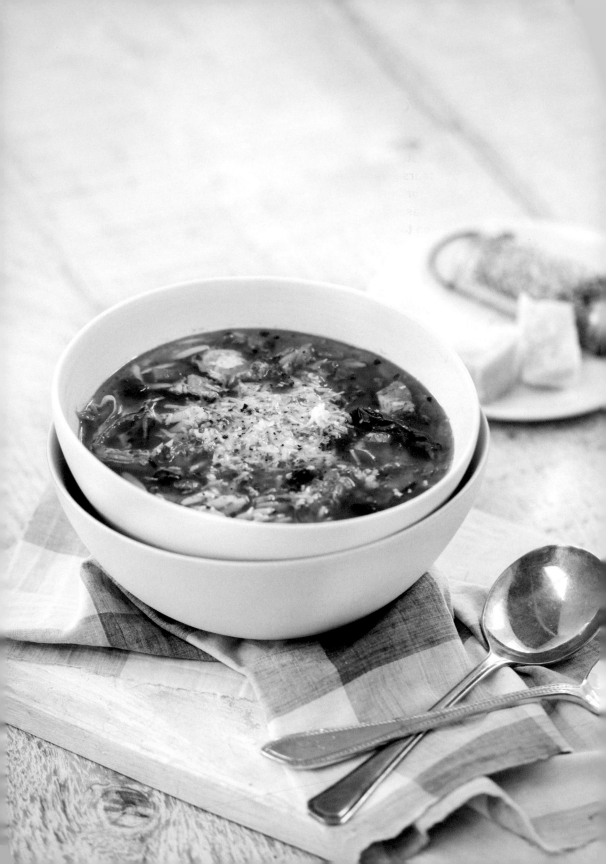

My Marvellous Minestrone Soup

I love to cook huge vats of this soup in true mamma Italiana style. This recipe is for four but, of course, you can double or triple it and keep some, minus the pasta, in the fridge for another day (if you leave the pasta in, it will become too soft). If you have a basil plant hanging around on your windowsill, pop a few fresh basil leaves on top for an extra dimension – it will make you feel like a true Italian.

Serves 4	7g FAT	2.2g SATURATES	8.1g SUGARS	1.41g SALT	169 CALORIES

1 tablespoon olive oil

1 onion, peeled and
finely chopped

1 garlic clove, peeled
and crushed

2 rashers of back bacon, all
visible fat removed, chopped

2 carrots, peeled and finely diced

3 celery sticks, finely diced

½ red pepper, finely diced

1 courgette, finely diced

1 teaspoon tomato purée

1.25 litres beef, chicken or
vegetable stock

½ teaspoon dried oregano

salt and freshly ground black
pepper

100g cooked small pasta shapes

a handful of finely sliced spinach

a handful of chopped cabbage

4 tablespoons freshly grated
Parmesan cheese

Put the oil into a large heavy-based saucepan and gently fry the onion and garlic until soft but not coloured. Add the bacon, carrot, celery, pepper and courgette and fry until lightly browned.

Stir in the tomato purée, followed by the stock and oregano and season with salt and pepper. Bring to the boil, reduce to a simmer and cook, covered, until the vegetables are just soft.

Stir in the cooked pasta shapes with the spinach and cabbage and simmer until the leaves have wilted. Sprinkle the Parmesan on top to serve.

Cumin-Spiced Carrot and Butternut Squash Soup

Wow! This soup is brilliant on so many levels. It has a great vibrant orange colour, lots of fabulous spices and it's packed full of superfoods. This is a real favourite of mine on a cold winter's day, served with hunks of soda bread. You can, if you fancy, dry-fry some pumpkin and sunflower seeds to garnish this – not only will they look lovely, but they provide an extra bit of protein and a whack of those good-for-you fats that make your hair shine and skin gleam.

Serves 4 | 4g FAT | 0.5g SATURATES | 20.4g SUGARS | 0.62g SALT | 199 CALORIES

1 tablespoon olive oil
1 onion, peeled and finely chopped
3 garlic cloves, peeled and finely chopped or crushed
1 red chilli (optional), deseeded if preferred, and chopped
1 teaspoon ground cumin
½ teaspoon ground ginger
500g carrots, peeled and cut into chunks
1 medium butternut squash, peeled and cubed
1 litre chicken or vegetable stock
1 teaspoon whole cumin seeds
1–2 tablespoons finely chopped fresh coriander, to garnish

Heat the oil in a large heavy-based saucepan and gently fry the onion until soft but not coloured, then add the garlic and chilli (if using) and give it all a good stir. Sprinkle in the ground cumin and ginger and stir well to release their aromas. Throw in the carrots and butternut squash, pour in the stock and bring up to the boil. Cover and simmer gently for about 10 minutes until the vegetables are cooked and tender.

Meanwhile, dry-fry the cumin seeds in a small pan to release their aroma. Pour the soup into a blender and blitz until smooth. To serve, ladle into soup bowls, sprinkle the toasted cumin seeds over the top and scatter over the fresh coriander.

'Try not to reward yourself with food – it will end up feeling like a punishment when you can't get your zip up!'

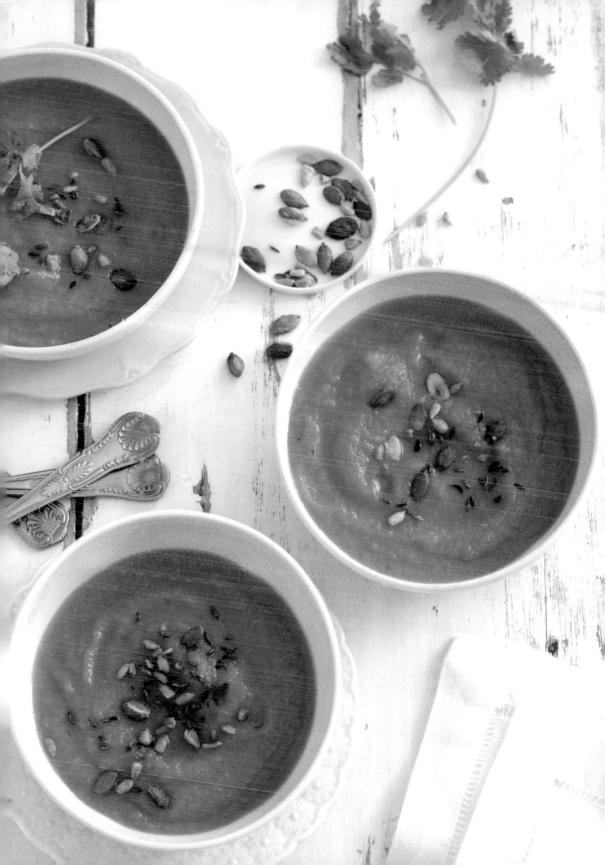

Spectacular Sandwiches

I'm not a fan of shop-bought sandwiches, but there's good reason for this. Just take a look at the average calorie and fat content and you'll see it can equal that of fish and chips – and, to be quite honest, I know which one I prefer!

So, let's talk about what makes a good sandwich. Firstly, they have to be quick and easy to make. Secondly, they have to look and taste delicious. And thirdly, they have to give you the power and energy to function well until dinnertime. I want my sandwiches packed full of luscious ingredients and always with some form of protein – because that's what keeps away the hunger pangs and helps build muscle. As a great man or woman (probably woman) once said, 'if you don't have a plan, you plan to fail'. So if I know I'm going to be out at work all day, I will put together a fabulous sandwich to take with me.

New York Deli-Style Sandwich

Now, I call this a New York Deli 'style' sandwich because a traditional New York deli sandwich is made with pastrami but, because pastrami is so calorie-dense, I have swapped it for smoked turkey so that us greedy girls can have lots and lots more filling! With the mayo mustard and pickles, it feels like the naughtiest sandwich in the world.

Serves 1	6.9g FAT	1.2g SATURATES	6.2g SUGARS	2.78g SALT	348 CALORIES

2 slices of pumpernickel bread
1 teaspoon American mustard
1 tablespoon light mayo
5 slices of thinly sliced
   smoked turkey
1 gherkin, sliced
1 tomato, sliced
a handful of shredded lettuce

Lightly toast the bread and spread with the mustard and mayo. Pile on the remaining ingredients and feast like a true American!

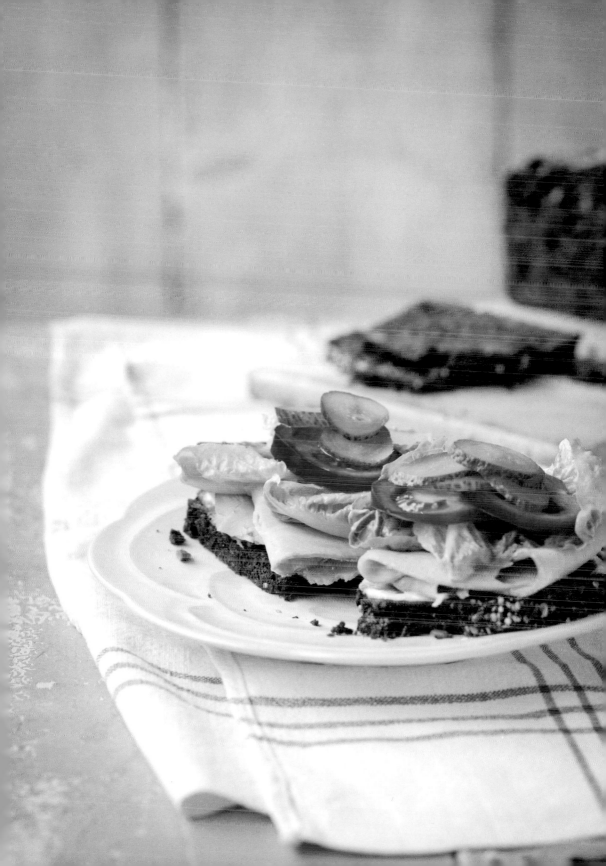

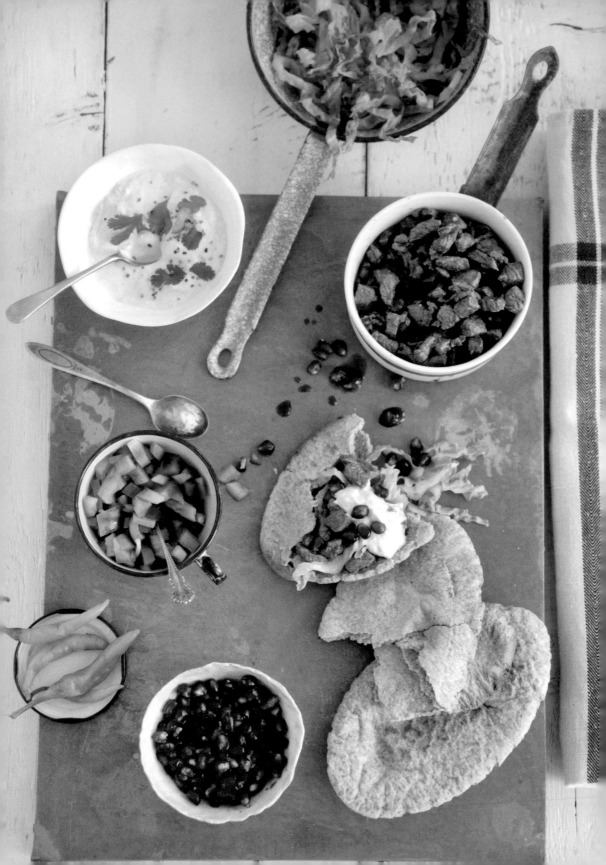

Spicy Lamb and Hummus Pitta

This is a sandwich that I make if I have a couple of girlfriends popping round for a quick lunch. It's a bit more fancy than a work sandwich, but still very easy to make and packed full of really tasty ingredients. Treat yourself!

Serves 4 | 5g FAT | 1.5g SATURATES | 4.9g SUGARS | 0.99g SALT | 228 CALORIES

100g lean lamb, cut into tiny
  pieces
1 garlic clove, peeled
  and crushed
1 teaspoon baharat spice blend
freshly ground black pepper
4 tablespoons reduced-fat
  hummus
1 tablespoon lemon juice
3 tablespoons water
2 tablespoons chopped fresh
  coriander
olive oil spray
4 wholemeal pitta breads
a small cos lettuce, finely
  chopped
1 green pepper, finely chopped
4 tablespoons pomegranate
  seeds

To serve
4 pickled green chilli peppers

Put the chopped lamb in a bowl, add the garlic, baharat spice blend and some black pepper and mix well together. Cover and set aside to marinate in the fridge for a couple of hours or, if possible, overnight. If you don't have the time, you can cook the lamb straight away and it will still be delicious.

Meanwhile, in a small bowl, combine the hummus with the lemon juice, 3 tablespoons water and the coriander. Beat until smooth and set aside.

Heat a non-stick frying pan sprayed with oil and fry the lamb over a medium heat until just browned, stirring constantly; set aside. Heat the pitta breads and open them.

To assemble the sarnies, stuff the pitta breads first with lettuce and then with some green pepper. Top with the lamb and drizzle over the hummus mixture. Finish with a flourish of pomegranate seeds. Serve with a pickled chilli on the side.

Salad Niçoise Sandwiches

Salad Niçoise is a great French classic that works just as well as a sandwich. Compare all these gorgeous ingredients to a limp tuna and cucumber sandwich you might expect to buy in a shop – no comparison.

Serves 4	8g FAT	1.7g SATURATES	4.4g SUGARS	1.21g SALT	308 CALORIES

2 x 200g cans of tuna in
   springwater
½ red onion, peeled and
   finely chopped
4 tablespoons finely chopped
   green or red pepper
4 tablespoons canned sweetcorn
2 tablespoons chopped fresh
   flat-leaf parsley
a few fresh basil leaves
8 black or green pitted olives,
   chopped
1 tablespoon olive oil
a big squeeze of lemon juice
freshly ground black pepper
2 small hard-boiled eggs
4 wholemeal pitta breads

Combine the tuna, red onion, pepper, sweetcorn, parsley, basil and olives in a large bowl. Drizzle over the olive oil and lemon juice, season with black pepper and give it all a good stir.

Chop up the boiled eggs and gently fold them in. Pile the mixture into warmed pitta bread, or serve on a plate with the pitta bread on the side.

'Pause for a moment before you eat something you probably shouldn't and ask yourself whether what you really want is a hug. Emotional hunger cannot be satisfied with food.'

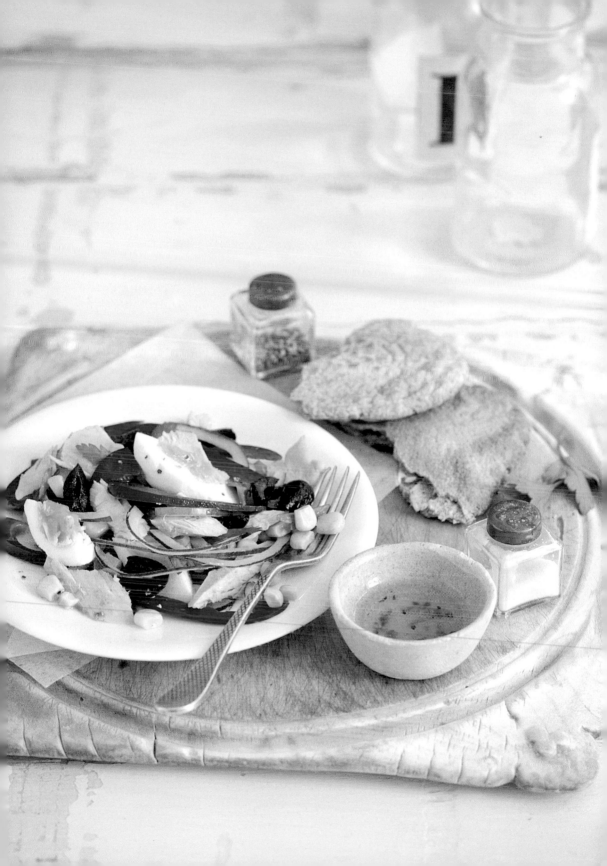

Chicken Lettuce Wraps

Whenever I feel as if I've been eating too much bread, I love to make these lettuce wraps – and so do the kids. Sometimes I swap the strips of chicken for lean beef or cooked prawns, and noodles for the rice. See which you like best!

Serves 1   11g FAT | 2.7g SATURATES | 13g SUGARS | 1.25g SALT | 364 CALORIES

2 large iceberg lettuce leaves
1 cooked skinless chicken
   breast, cut into thin strips
3 tablespoons cooked brown rice
½ green pepper, cut into thin strips
1 carrot, peeled and cut into
   thin strips

For the sauce
2 teaspoons peanut butter
2 teaspoons hot water
1 teaspoon soy sauce

In a small bowl, mix together the ingredients for the sauce and set aside.

Lay out the lettuce leaves on a work surface and divide the chicken, rice, pepper and carrot between them. Drizzle over the peanut sauce, roll up the lettuce leaves and voilà! Super delicious, super easy, Chinesey chicken lettuce wraps.

Peanut Butter Power-Packed Lunch

You may look at these ingredients and think I'm mad but, trust me, they all go together brilliantly. The Marmite and peanut butter give a wonderful sweet and salty flavour, while the alfalfa and cucumber really freshen things up. I sometimes have this sandwich for breakfast as well as lunch!

Serves 1   9g FAT | 1.8g SATURATES | 2.5g SUGARS | 1.37g SALT | 226 CALORIES

2 slices rye or wholemeal bread
Marmite, for spreading
1 tablespoon peanut, almond or
   cashew butter
large handful of alfalfa sprouts
sliced cucumber

Spread the slices of bread with Marmite and top with the peanut butter.

Pile on the alfalfa and as much cucumber as you fancy, and sandwich together.

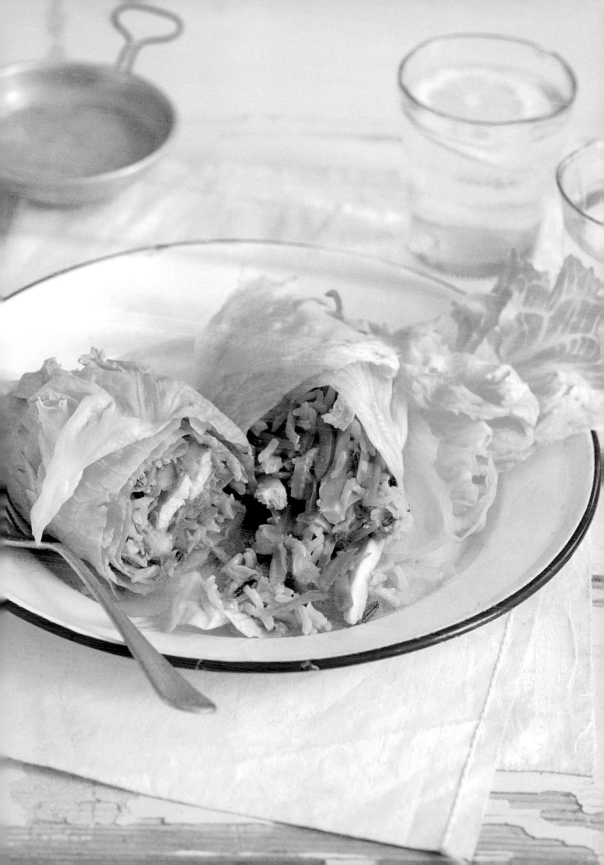

Super-Duper Salads

Traditionally, we tend to think of salads in this country as a penance, a brutal punishment for being on the lardy side, but I most definitely don't. To me, they're a source of great pleasure with which I can get really creative. One of the mistakes that can be made with salads is simply not putting enough in the bowl. On this one, we need to look to the Americans, who serve their salads in washing-up bowl sized dishes. The second mistake that's often made when people are watching their weight and eating salads is that they omit all oil from the salad. Don't do this or you'll end up with a rather tasteless salad and a depressing sense of injustice. Just be sure to measure carefully HOW MUCH oil you put in. On hungrier days, feel free to add some extra protein (like cooked chicken or tinned tuna) or some extra carbs (maybe a slice of rye toast or some boiled new potatoes). Come on ladies – let's celebrate the salad!

Carrot and Mouli Salad

This is a great alternative to traditional, fattier, coleslaw, and because of the added cumin, it would go really well with lamb. I also like it alongside my Za'atar Chicken (page 96). To make this into a main meal, serving two, bulk it up by scattering pumpkin seeds and sunflower seeds on top.

Serves 4 as a side salad, or 2 as a main (nutritional values given for dish as a side salad)

5g FAT | 0.6g SATURATES | 5.2g SUGARS | 0.08g SALT | 73 CALORIES

200g carrots, peeled and coarsely grated

200g mouli, peeled and coarsely grated

salt

1½ tablespoons lime juice

1½ tablespoons sunflower oil

1 tablespoon cumin seeds

Put the grated carrots and mouli into a bowl, season with salt and mix well. Add the lime juice and combine thoroughly.

Heat the sunflower oil in a frying pan over a medium heat, throw in the cumin seeds and swirl them around in the pan until they start popping. Pour the oil and seeds over the salad and stir well.

Mackerel with Horseradish, Rocket and Beetroot Salad and Rye Toast

Wow, what a treat of a lunch this is – one that you deserve and one that won't take you more than five minutes to put together. It's very pretty to look at and the oily fish will help make YOU very pretty to look at, because all those great fish oils are fantastic for your hair and skin.

Serves 4 | 20g FAT | 5.1g SATURATES | 7.7g SUGARS | 1.92g SALT | 281 CALORIES

2 cooked beetroots, cubed
1 cooked small potato, cubed
handful of salad leaves
4 tomatoes, diced
250g smoked mackerel fillet

For the dressing
1 teaspoon creamed horseradish
1 tablespoon low-fat crème
   fraîche
1 teaspoon chopped gherkin

To serve
4 slices of rye bread, toasted
4 handfuls of rocket

To make the dressing, combine the horseradish, crème fraîche and gherkin in a bowl. Add the cubed beetroot and potato and stir well to coat them in the dressing.

Arrange the salad leaves on a plate, scatter over the tomatoes and flake over the mackerel. Finish with a handful of rocket leaves, and serve with the beetroot and potato salad and a slice of toasted rye bread on the side.

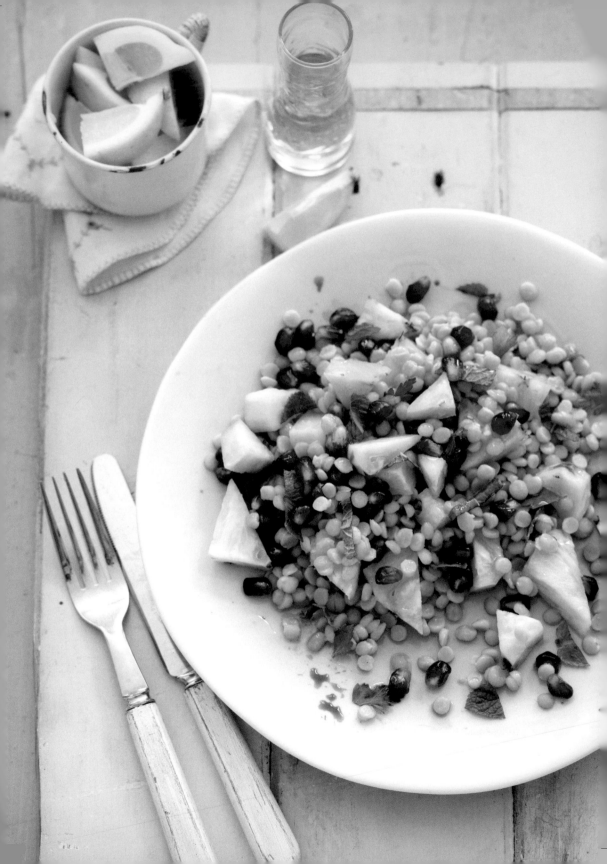

Sunshine Salad

The bright colours and fresh flavours in this delicious salad really do feel like a burst of brilliant sunshine on your plate.

Serves 4	7g FAT	0.8g SATURATES	8.5g SUGARS	0.05g SALT	255 CALORIES

180g yellow lentils
½ teaspoon ground turmeric
1 tablespoon lemon juice
2 tablespoons olive oil
salt
seeds of ½ pomegranate
75g diced pineapple
4 tablespoons finely chopped
    fresh flat-leaf parsley
4 tablespoons finely chopped
    fresh mint

Put the lentils into a saucepan with 700ml water and the turmeric, bring to the boil and then simmer, covered, for about 20 minutes until tender. Keep an eye on them after 10 minutes to make sure they don't turn into a mush. Drain and turn into a bowl.

While the lentils are still warm, stir in the lemon juice and oil, adding a little salt. Set aside to cool.

To assemble the salad, stir in the rest of the ingredients and serve.

Spice up your Sardines

Sardines are just too good for us to be ignored, so I've helped them along by spicing them up a little. I promise you, this is a delicious way to eat them!

Serves 4	13g FAT	2.8g SATURATES	2.2g SUGARS	1.44g SALT	253 CALORIES

olive oil spray
1 garlic clove, peeled and crushed
½ teaspoon chopped red chilli
a squeeze of lemon juice
4 slices of rye or granary bread
4 x 120g cans of sardines in
    tomato sauce
1 teaspoon finely chopped fresh
    flat-leaf parsley

Fry the garlic and chilli in olive oil spray over a low heat for a few minutes until soft. Squeeze in the lemon juice and remove from the heat.

Meanwhile, toast the bread and arrange the sardines on top. Sprinkle the garlic and chilli mixture on top of the sardines and garnish with chopped parsley. Serve this with a massive salad and you will feel like a saint!

Chicken and Avocado Salad

Although avocados are high in fat, it's mono-saturated fat – which is the good kind! (Thank the lord as they are so delicious it would be a shame to carry the guilt!) They also contain even more potassium than bananas, and lots of vitamins. This salad includes chicken, crispy bacon and walnuts – so many delicious flavours and textures, you'll hardly feel like it's a salad at all!

Serves 4	35g FAT	5.9g SATURATES	1.3g SUGARS	1.03g SALT	513 CALORIES

4 rashers of back bacon with fat removed, finely chopped

1 large bag of baby leaf spinach

4 cooked skinless chicken breasts, cut into thin strips

1 avocado, stoned and cut into rough chunks

16 walnuts, halved

a handful of fresh flat-leaf parsley, finely chopped

For the dressing
1 teaspoon Dijon mustard
½ shallot, peeled and finely chopped
salt and freshly ground black pepper
3 tablespoons rice vinegar
2 tablespoons olive oil

Dry-fry the bacon until crisp, then drain on kitchen paper and set aside. Put the spinach leaves into a large bowl with the chicken, avocado and walnuts.

To make the dressing, put the mustard and shallot into a small bowl with some salt and pepper and whisk in the vinegar and olive oil.

Drizzle the dressing over the salad, sprinkle with the chopped parsley and divide equally between 4 plates. Finish off by scattering the bacon on top.

'Don't beat yourself up. If you have a lapse, please don't hit the self-destruct button and start eating everything again. Just refocus on your goal ASAP.'

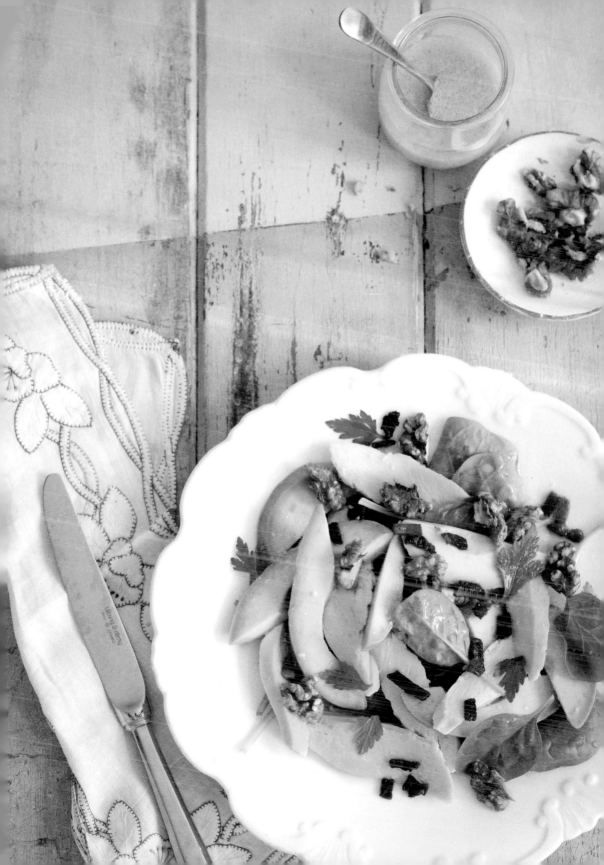

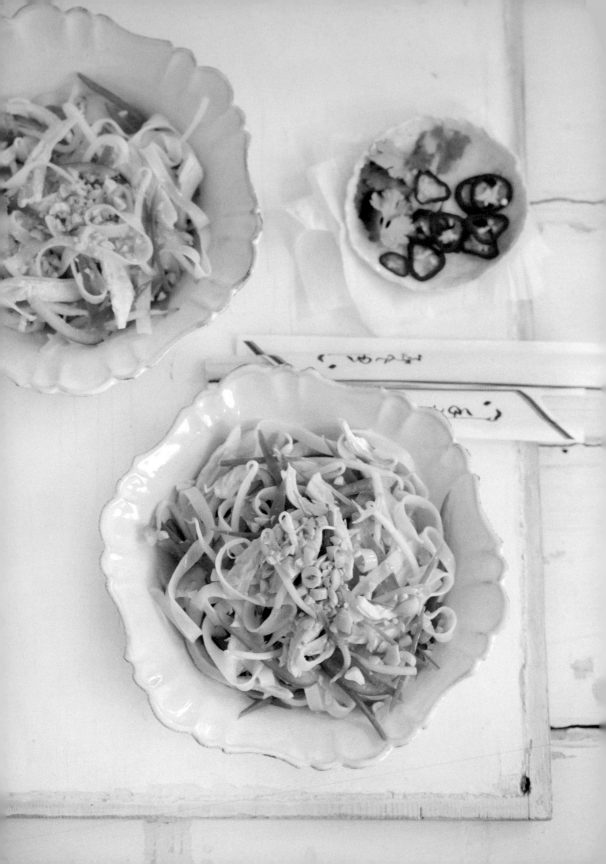

Chilli Chicken Noodle Salad

This salad is such a treat! It's really flavoursome and feels ever so naughty, but I promise you there is no sin in it. You can swap the chicken for prawns if you wish or, if you're a vegetarian (or just mad enough to like tofu) you can use some tofu instead.

Serves 4	12g FAT	2.4g SATURATES	5g SUGARS	0.94g SALT	419 CALORIES

200g dried thin rice noodles

4 small chicken breasts, cooked and shredded

2 carrots, peeled and cut into very thin matchsticks

a handful of beansprouts

1 green pepper, cut into very thin strips

For the dressing

2 tablespoons sesame oil

1 tablespoon fish sauce

1 tablespoon lime juice

a pinch of sugar

1 fresh red chilli (deseeded, if preferred)

To garnish

1 tablespoon crushed peanuts

2 tablespoons chopped fresh coriander

Cook the noodles according to packet instructions, drain well and place in a large salad bowl. Add the shredded chicken to the bowl along with the carrot, beansprouts and green pepper.

To make the dressing, combine all the dressing ingredients in a small bowl and whisk until smooth.

To serve, drizzle the dressing over the noodles, toss well and top with the peanuts and coriander.

Beetroot and Potato Salad

Liven up the humble potato salad by adding a splash of colour with lovely red beetroot, and the tangy bite of pickled dill cucumber.

Serves 4 as a side salad

6g FAT | 1.1g SATURATES | 13.5g SUGARS | 0.48g SALT | 179 CALORIES

250g waxy potatoes, scrubbed
500g cooked beetroot (without
    vinegar), cut into 1cm cubes
1 small pickled dill cucumber
a handful of chopped fresh dill,
    plus some sprigs, to garnish
½ teaspoon dried dill (optional)
approx. 4 heaped tablespoons
    low-fat Greek yogurt

For the vinaigrette dressing
1 tablespoon balsamic vinegar
2 tablespoons sunflower oil
½ teaspoon French mustard
2 medium garlic cloves, peeled
    and finely chopped

Steam or boil the potatoes in their skins, then drain and cut into 1cm cubes. To make the dressing, whisk all the dressing ingredients in a small bowl. Combine the potatoes in a salad bowl with the diced beetroot. Stir in enough of the dressing to coat the vegetables nicely and set aside to cool.

Meanwhile, chop the dill cucumber into small pieces and finely chop the fresh dill. Stir the cucumber, fresh dill and dried dill (if using) into the potato and beetroot mixture.

When you are ready to serve, stir in the Greek yogurt. (Don't do this too soon, because the yogurt will sink into the beetroot and then it won't be very pretty). Decorate with sprigs of fresh dill.

Carrot Salad

Serves 4 as a side salad

0.3g FAT | 0.0g SATURATES | 7.6g SUGARS | 0.06g SALT | 36 CALORIES

400g organic carrots
salt, to taste
juice of 1 lemon

Peel and finely grate the carrots and place them in a salad bowl. Season to taste, stir in the lemon juice and serve.

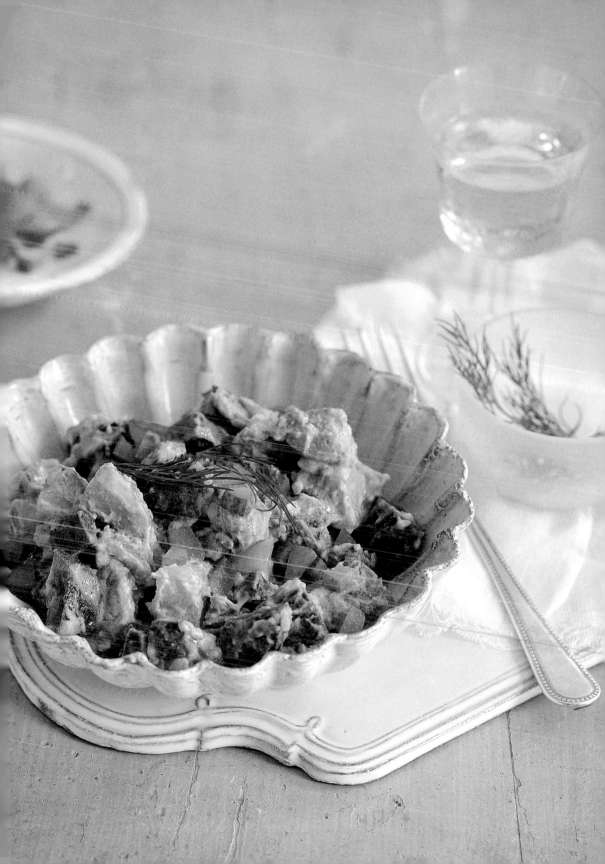

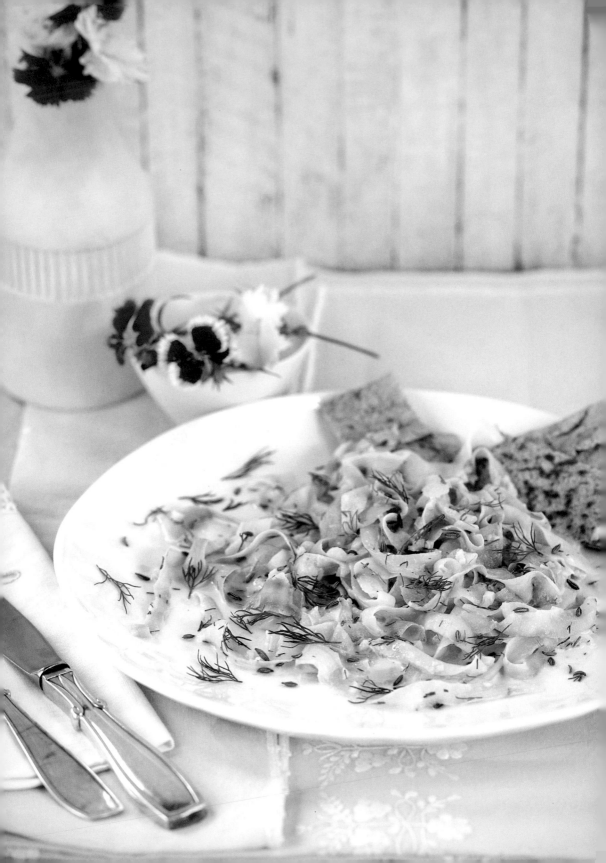

Cucumber Salad

I love to serve this salad alongside grilled white fish for supper or as a main course for lunch with some warm pitta breads. It also works really well as a filling for jacket potatoes.

Serves 4 as a side salad

1g FAT | 0.1g SATURATES | 1.7g SUGARS | 0.53g SALT | 20 CALORIES

1 cucumber

1 teaspoon salt

½ tablespoon cider vinegar

½ tablespoon dill vinegar from a jar of dill cucumbers (or 2 teaspoons cider vinegar mixed with ½ teaspoon water, if you have no dill vinegar)

3 tablespoons chopped fresh dill, plus a few sprigs, to garnish

1 tablespoon very finely chopped shallot or spring onion

1½ tablespoons low-fat crème fraîche, soured cream or yogurt

½ tablespoon dill seeds

Peel the cucumber and slice it very thinly. Put in a colander, sprinkle with the salt and toss with your hands to distribute the salt evenly. Rinse, and then set aside to drain for 10 minutes.

Put the drained cucumber into a bowl. Combine the vinegars in a separate bowl and stir in the chopped dill. Pour the mixture over the cucumber and stir in the chopped shallot (or spring onion) and crème fraîche (or soured cream or yogurt). Arrange on a flat serving dish, sprinkle over the dill seeds and decorate with a few dill fronds.

Chicory, Orange and Walnut Salad

Chicory is a very underused leaf and I think this is because it has a reputation for being bitter, so ensure you buy the ones with a yellow hue; the green ones are the naughty ones with a bitter taste!

Serves 4 as a side salad

20g FAT | 5.5g SATURATES | 5.5g SUGARS | 2.11g SALT | 269 CALORIES

1 orange
1 head of chicory, sliced into
    2cm rounds
3 tablespoons chopped walnuts
1 x 225g packet of light halloumi
    cheese, cut into thick slices
olive oil spray

For the dressing
2 teaspoons sherry vinegar
8 teaspoons walnut oil
½ teaspoon French mustard
1 medium garlic clove, peeled
    and very finely chopped
salt

Peel the orange and cut into small pieces on a plate to catch the juices. Strain the juice into a small bowl and whisk in the dressing ingredients.

Place the chicory, orange pieces and walnuts in a salad bowl and pour over the dressing.

Spray the halloumi slices with olive oil and griddle on a hot pan until golden brown on each side. Scatter over the salad and serve.

Lily's Noodle Salad

This is my Auntie Lily's recipe. She is Chinese, so she knows what she is talking about when it comes to noodles! You could add some shredded cooked chicken or tofu to the salad if you wish – and some chilli sauce will add a bit of a kick, if you fancy that!

Serves 4   6g FAT | 0.9g SATURATES | 1.8g SUGARS | 2.81g SALT | 352 CALORIES

300g cellophane noodles
500g baby leaf spinach
2 tablespoons chopped fresh
   coriander
2 tablespoons finely sliced
   spring onions
1 medium garlic clove, peeled
   and finely chopped
300g tofu or cooked chicken,
   shredded (optional)

For the dressing
3 tablespoons soy sauce
1½ tablespoons toasted
   sesame oil
½ teaspoon salt
½ teaspoon sugar

Drop the noodles into a large saucepan of boiling water and cook for 20 minutes. While the noodles are cooking, whisk together the ingredients for the dressing.

Drain the noodles and cut into shorter lengths with scissors (otherwise, they are difficult to serve). Place in a serving bowl. While the noodles are still hot, stir in the spinach, fresh coriander, spring onion and garlic. Pour over the dressing and top with the tofu or cooked chicken, if you are indulging!

Ladies Who Lunch

This section is all about those rare days when we have a bit of time to stop, socialise and enjoy some good food in good company.

Spicy Chick Pea Tagine

This is one of those great dishes you can cook the day before, allowing the flavours to develop and making it even tastier to indulge in. It's extremely cheap to make and a juicy lamb chop would go perfectly alongside it.

Serves 4	7g FAT	0.8g SATURATES	6.7g SUGARS	0.55g SALT	173 CALORIES

2 tablespoons olive oil
2 onions, peeled and sliced
4 garlic cloves, peeled and cut into quarters
1 teaspoon ground cumin
1 teaspoon ground cinnamon
1 cinnamon stick
1 teaspoon ground coriander
1 teaspoon ground turmeric
1 x 400g can whole plum tomatoes
200ml chicken stock
1 x 400g can chick peas, drained
salt and freshly ground black pepper

Heat the oil in a heavy-based pan and fry the onion and garlic until soft. Add all the spices and stir for a minute to release their aromas.

Now add the tomatoes (left whole) and the stock. Bring to the boil, and then reduce the heat and simmer for 40 minutes. Add the chick peas and simmer for a further 15 minutes.

Season with salt and pepper and serve. This is delicious with brown basmati rice and salad.

Spinach and Hazelnut Spaghetti

What could be more perfect than bunging a few divine ingredients into a food processor, blitzing them and stirring them into a big, comforting bowl of hot pasta? Read on...

Serves 4	25g FAT	3.1g SATURATES	4.1g SUGARS	0.12g SALT	590 CALORIES

400g spaghetti
½ garlic clove, peeled
50g baby leaf spinach
50g fresh basil leaves
100g roasted hazelnuts
20g freshly grated Parmesan
    cheese
2 tablespoons olive oil
salt and freshly ground black
    pepper

Cook the spaghetti according to packet instructions.

Meanwhile, make the spinach and hazelnut pesto. Put the garlic, three quarters of the spinach and the basil in a food processor and blitz until smooth, then add the hazelnuts and pulse a few times to give a coarse texture (rather than turning the mixture to mush). Spoon the mixture into a bowl and stir in the Parmesan and olive oil. Season with salt and pepper.

Drain the spaghetti and return to the pan. Tip in the spinach and hazelnut pesto and combine thoroughly. Serve garnished with the reserved spinach leaves.

'Don't leave leftovers lying around. Get them covered up and in the fridge or freezer straight away – then you won't be tempted to scoff the lot later!'

Broccoli, Mushroom and Chilli Parmesan Pasta

This is another really easy dish to make. As broccoli practically has a god-like status in the superfood hall of fame, we can feel quite saintly about eating it.

Now, I have stated in this recipe to use wholewheat pasta but, of course, if you can't bear it, just use white pasta. What I would say, however, is that brown pasta definitely keeps me fuller for longer. Believe me, in the name of science I have sacrificed myself countless times to bring you this data by devouring and comparing endless bowls of white AND brown pasta.

Serves 4	9g FAT	1.9g SATURATES	3.9g SUGARS	0.34g SALT	338 CALORIES

300g wholewheat pasta

250g broccoli, cut into florets

2 tablespoons olive oil

200g mushrooms, quartered

½ red chilli (deseeded if preferred), chopped

1 garlic clove, peeled and crushed or chopped

freshly ground black pepper

a little freshly grated Parmesan cheese

Cook the pasta according to packet instructions.

Meanwhile, steam the broccoli for a few minutes until just tender, drain and refresh under cold running water.

Heat the oil in a large frying pan and throw in the mushrooms. Stir over a medium heat for a minute or so until the mushrooms soften and then add the chilli and garlic and stir for another minute. Drain the pasta and tip it into the frying pan along with the broccoli. Toss everything together to mix and season with lots of freshly ground black pepper and a little Parmesan.

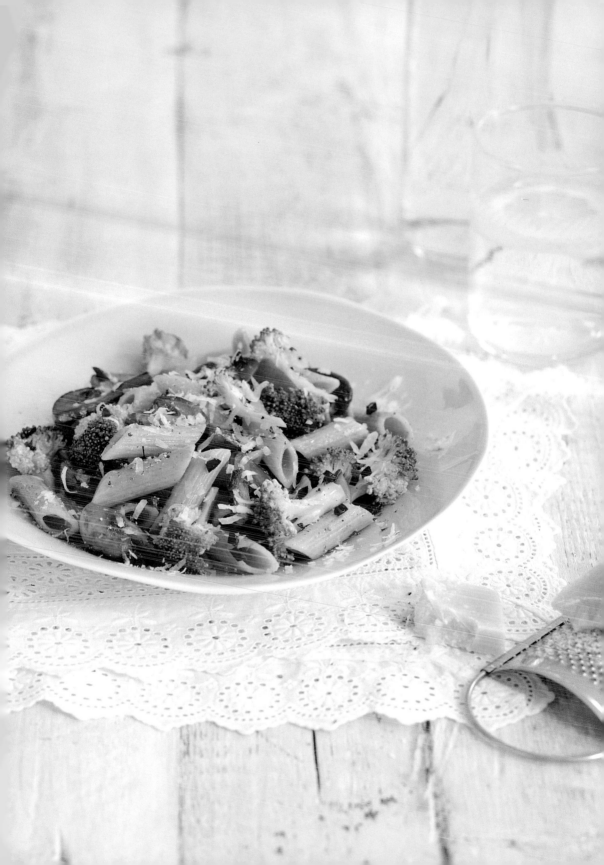

Chilli Lemon Tiger Prawns

I have to confess I'm a bit of a sweet chilli sauce addict and I'm always looking for new ways to satisfy my addiction – this recipe does it rather beautifully.

Serves 4	0.4g FAT	0.1g SATURATES	4.4g SUGARS	0.64g SALT	65 CALORIES

4 tablespoons lemon juice
1 tablespoon grated lemon zest
1 red chilli (deseeded if
    preferred), finely chopped
2 tablespoons sweet chilli sauce
salt
500g raw shell-on tiger prawns

Put the lemon juice, zest, chilli and sweet chilli sauce into a bowl and stir. Add a little salt, then toss the prawns in the mixture and set aside to marinate for half an hour or so.

To cook the prawns, either grill under a moderate heat until pink or – my absolute favourite – cook on a barbecue. Serve with a huge green salad and a fingerbowl.

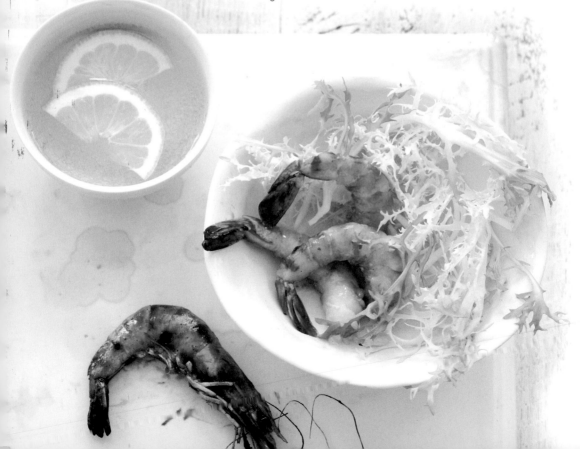

Spaghetti with Chilli, Crab and Lemon

This classic recipe is light, summery and incredibly easy to make. You can, of course, if you're lucky enough to get it, use fresh crabmeat instead of canned. Once again, I urge you to use wholewheat spaghetti rather than white.

Serves 4	8g FAT	1.1g SATURATES	4.5g SUGARS	0.86g SALT	382 CALORIES

350g wholewheat spaghetti
2 tablespoons olive oil
4 garlic cloves, peeled and
    finely chopped
1 red chilli (deseeded if
    preferred), finely chopped
1 x 200g can crabmeat, drained
½ glass white wine
a large handful of fresh flat-leaf
    parsley, chopped
zest of 1 large unwaxed lemon
a big squeeze of lemon juice
freshly ground black pepper

Cook the spaghetti according to packet instructions.

Heat the oil in a large frying pan and fry the garlic and chilli until soft but not coloured. Add the crabmeat and white wine and bring to the boil. Simmer for 1 minute, stirring.

Drain the spaghetti and tip it into the pan with the crab mixture. Add the parsley, the lemon zest and juice and season with black pepper. Give everything a good stir and serve with a rocket salad.

'Without wishing to sound like your mother, never eat standing up! You'd be amazed how many more calories you consume while standing and stuffing without realising it. Sit down and savour!'

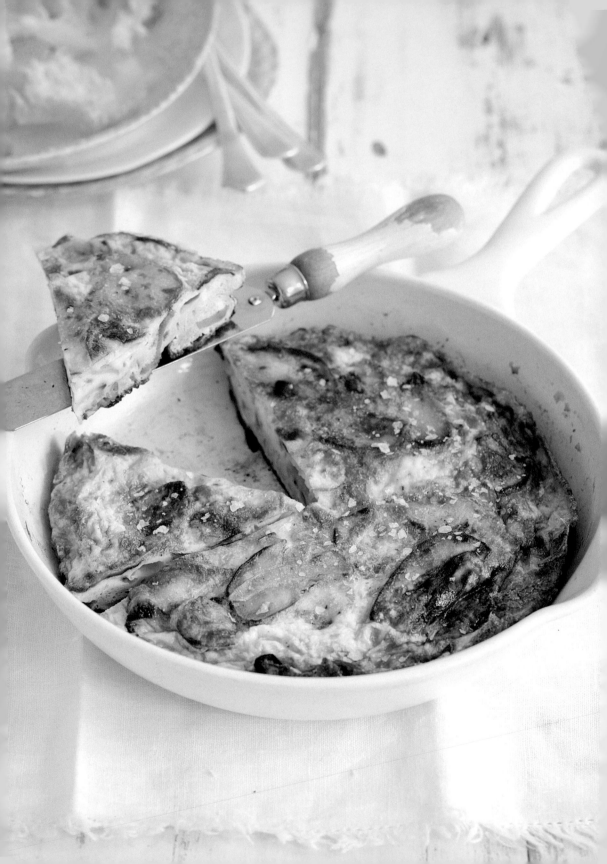

Spanish Tortilla

Now I bet you didn't expect to see Spanish tortilla in a book with 'diet' on the front cover, did you? But hey, we're greedy girls and we love lots of potatoes, so there's no way I was gonna miss it out. I would strongly advise that whenever you prepare the Spanish tortilla for you and friends, make sure you serve it with a cold crisp salad and a cold crisp glass of white wine beside it. You could make double the amount because It's just as lovely cold, and then you've got packed lunch sorted for the next day.

Serves 4	19g FAT	4.4g SATURATES	3.4g SUGARS	0.44g SALT	288 CALORIES

2 tablespoons olive oil

2 medium potatoes, peeled (if you wish) and very thinly and evenly sliced (I use a mandolin to do this)

1 large onion, peeled and thinly sliced

8 large eggs

salt and freshly ground black pepper

Heat the oil in a deep non-stick frying pan over a medium heat. Throw in the potatoes and gently fry for 5 minutes. Add the onion and cook, stirring the whole time, until soft and slightly browned.

Whisk the eggs, season with salt and pepper and pour into the frying pan. Cook over a medium heat for a couple of minutes and then, using a palette knife, draw the cooked egg into the middle and let the liquid egg run into the gaps. When the egg is set, put a plate over the pan and flip the omelette onto it. Slide the omelette back into the pan to cook to your taste on the other side

This tortilla is delicious hot or cold with a crisp salad and, if my mum has anything to do with it, a glass of cold white wine!

Family Sunday Lunch

These recipes are all about those times when we can relax a little in the kitchen, turn on some music, maybe pop open a bottle of wine and spend a bit longer cooking for ourselves and those we love – not too much wine, though, otherwise all the resolve will go out the window and you'll find yourself chomping on a bag of crisps... or six!

Beer Can Barbecued Chicken

This is such a nifty recipe, as the beer flavours and moistens the chicken from the inside whilst leaving the skin to become lovely and crispy. Now you will need a barbecue with a lid for this recipe, but if you don't have one it's lovely in the oven too. Just roast at 200°C/gas mark 6 for 1 hour and 10 minutes.

Serves 4	25g FAT	7.9g SATURATES	0.9g SUGARS	0.44g SALT	421 CALORIES

½ onion, peeled and finely chopped

1 garlic clove, peeled and crushed

1 teaspoon each of chopped fresh thyme and oregano

1 teaspoon paprika

salt and freshly ground black pepper

a large knob of light butter, melted

1.5kg whole chicken

1 x 440ml can lager

sprig of fresh thyme

you will need a vertical beer can chicken roasting stand (available online)

To make the marinade, combine the onion, garlic, herbs, paprika, salt and pepper in a bowl with the butter and give it all a good stir. Rub the marinade all over the chicken and set aside in the fridge to marinate for at least an hour, preferably overnight.

Pour the lager out of the can and set aside. Carefully cut the top off the can (it will be sharp!) and put in a sprig of thyme. Pour the beer back in, place the can in the middle of the roasting stand and mount the chicken on top. Loosely cover the top of the chicken with a piece of foil and transfer the stand to the barbie. Put on the lid and cook for 1½ –2 hours. To check the chicken is cooked, just pierce the thigh with a sharp knife – the juices should run clear. Remove the chicken carefully because the can will be extremely hot

Roasted Pork Meatballs in Tomato Sauce

Lots of people make the mistake of thinking that pork is a fatty meat. Actually, it's quite the opposite and, as long as you remove any of the visible fat, pork is incredibly lean. So, with that in mind, I've swapped the more traditional beef meatballs for pork meatballs. This is a nice dish to make if you have kids, because I haven't met a kid yet that doesn't like spaghetti and meatballs. They can also get stuck in and help you make them.

Serves 4 | 14g FAT | 3.4g SATURATES | 7.6g SUGARS | 0.33g SALT | 596 CALORIES

For the meatballs
a bunch of fresh flat-leaf parsley
1 onion, peeled and
   roughly chopped
500g lean minced pork
zest of 2 unwaxed lemons
salt and freshly ground black
   pepper
400g spaghetti

For the sauce
2 tablespoons olive oil
2 garlic cloves, peeled
   and crushed
70g tomato purée
1 teacup of boiling water
freshly grated Parmesan
   cheese, to serve

Preheat the oven to 200°C/gas mark 6. Put the parsley into a food processor and blitz until it's really finely chopped, then add the onion and whizz again. Add the pork and lemon zest and pulse until everything is beautifully mixed. Season.

To shape the meatballs, wet your hands (so that the meat doesn't stick to them) and roll the mixture into hazelnut-sized balls. Put them into a roasting tin and roast for 10 minutes until cooked through.

Meanwhile, cook the spaghetti according to packet instructions.

To make the sauce, heat the oil in a non-stick frying pan and fry the garlic very gently until soft but not coloured. Add the tomato purée and stir for a few minutes. Pour in the hot water and stir to combine, then turn off the heat. Drain the spaghetti, tip it into the frying pan and toss until evenly coated in the tomato sauce. Spoon the spaghetti into serving bowls, top with the meatballs and grate over some fresh Parmesan.

Herbed Pork Chops with Salted Baked Potatoes

This recipe is inspired by the flavours of Greece – plenty of herbs and brightly coloured peppers with rich olive oil, lemon and pork. I suggest that while cooking the pork chops you leave the fat on, but ensure you take it off just before serving. This way the pork is nice and juicy but not too calorific.

Serves 4	11g FAT	2.7g SATURATES	9.6g SUGARS	2.69g SALT	316 CALORIES

4 pork chops on the bone
juice of 1 lemon
2 garlic cloves, peeled
    and crushed
1 sprig each of fresh rosemary,
    oregano and thyme, finely
    chopped
salt and freshly ground black
    pepper
4 small baking potatoes
1 egg white, lightly beaten
2 tablespoons olive oil
2 onions, peeled and
    roughly sliced
1 red pepper, sliced
1 yellow pepper, sliced
1 green pepper, sliced
4–6 garlic cloves, peeled and
    crushed or chopped
a pinch of sugar

Preheat the oven to 200°C/gas mark 6.

Marinate the pork in the lemon juice, garlic, herbs and seasoning for at least an hour.

Dip the potatoes in the beaten egg white and roll in some salt. Bake in a roasting tin for 45 minutes.

Heat the oil in a frying pan, add the onion, peppers, garlic and sugar and fry gently until soft.

Place a griddle pan on the stove top and heat until very hot. Sear the pork chops until just browned on each side. Leave the fat on while the chops cook, but don't forget to remove it before serving! Now reduce the heat to low and cook for a further 8–10 minutes until the meat is cooked through – the time needed depends on the thickness of your pork. Please don't overcook the meat; it would be such a shame if the chops were to dry out. Serve with the gorgeous peppers and onions piled on top of the salted baked potatoes.

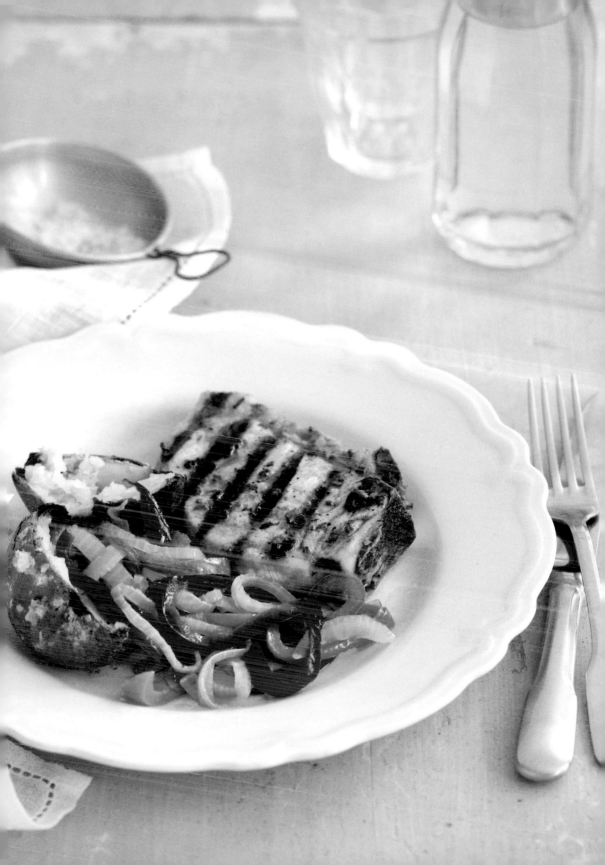

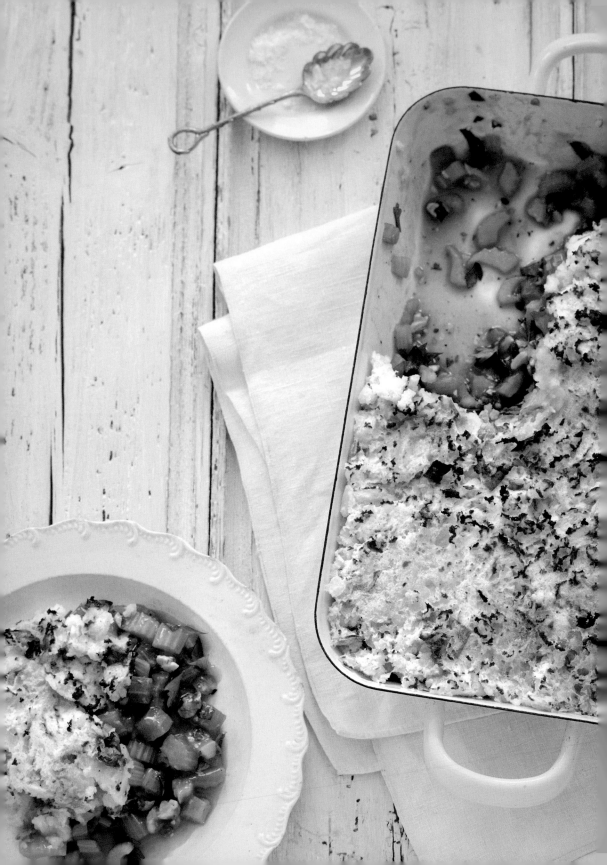

Vegetarian Comfort Pie

This is my sister's favourite Sunday dish and she always implores me to make it because she says it comforts her like nothing else does without any guilt!

Serves 4	1g FAT	0.1g SATURATES	4.1g SUGARS	0.57g SALT	145 CALORIES

1 large or 2 small bunches of
 celery, cut into 2cm cubes
300ml vegetable stock
a good slosh of brandy (you could
 use whisky if you don't have
 any brandy)
½–1 teaspoon Marmite,
 Vegemite or other
 vegetable extract
1 tablespoon cornflour mixed
 with 2 tablespoons cold water
salt and freshly ground black
 pepper

For the mash
500g potatoes, such as Lady
 Balfour, Maris Piper or Yukon
 Gold, peeled and chopped
150ml skimmed milk
a grating of nutmeg (optional)

Put the celery into a saucepan, pour over the stock and simmer for 15 minutes. Drain, reserving the stock in the pan.

Return the pan of stock to the heat, bring back to the boil and stir in the brandy, Marmite and plenty of freshly ground black pepper. Add the cornflour mixture and stir until the sauce thickens. Pour into an ovenproof casserole and stir in the celery. Place on the hob and simmer, covered, for 15 minutes.

Meanwhile, boil the potatoes in salted water until soft, then drain. Bring the milk to the boil in the same pan and add the grated nutmeg (if using). Tip in the potatoes, mash well and season with freshly ground black pepper.

Preheat the grill to high. Spread the mashed potato over the top of the celery mixture, fork them up and pop under the grill until they are nicely browned.

Za'atar Chicken

This is a Middle Eastern favourite of mine. Za'atar is a gorgeous blend of thyme, oregano, sumac and sesame seeds and it goes brilliantly with meat, fish or poultry. You can get it from Turkish or Middle Eastern shops. Try to track it down – you won't regret it!

Serves 4	8g FAT	2g SATURATES	6.6g SUGARS	1.03g SALT	316 CALORIES

8 skinless chicken pieces (a mixture of legs and thighs, on the bone)

For the marinade
4 garlic cloves, peeled and finely chopped
juice of 1 lemon
salt

2 large onions, peeled and roughly chopped
½ tablespoon za'atar (if you can't find za'atar, use dried thyme or oregano instead)
1–2 tablespoons olive oil mixed with ½ tablespoon za'atar (or thyme or oregano) and ½ teaspoon salt

First marinate the chicken. Lay the chicken pieces in a roasting tin. Combine the garlic with the lemon juice and salt, then pour the mixture over the chicken and set aside to marinate in the fridge for at least 2 hours.

Preheat the oven to 230°C/gas mark 8.

Remove the chicken from the roasting tin. Scatter the onion over the base of the tin, sprinkle with ½ tablespoon za'atar and arrange the chicken pieces on top. Brush the chicken with the oil mixture and roast in the oven for 10 minutes. Reduce the heat to 200°C/gas mark 6 and roast for a further 35 minutes or until cooked through.

Serve with a big mixed salad, or my Carrot and Mouli Salad (page 68).

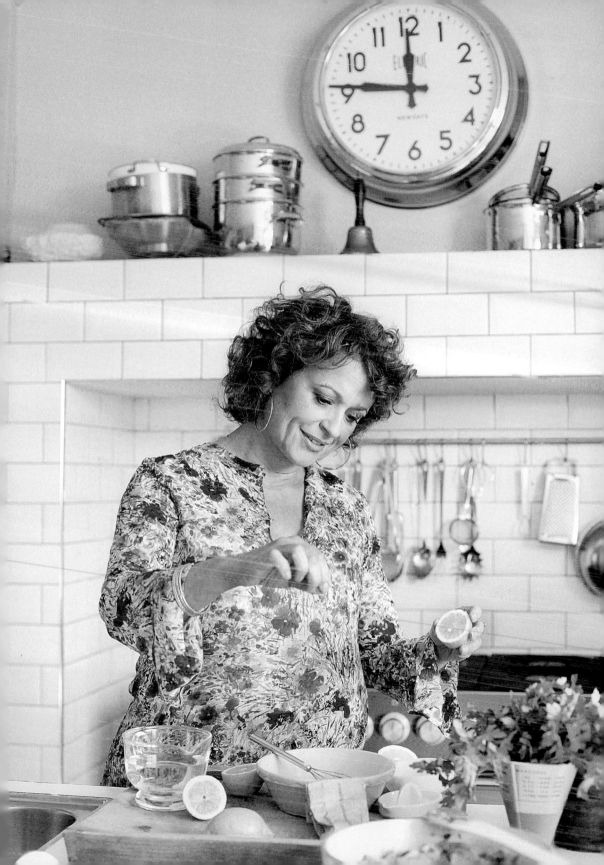

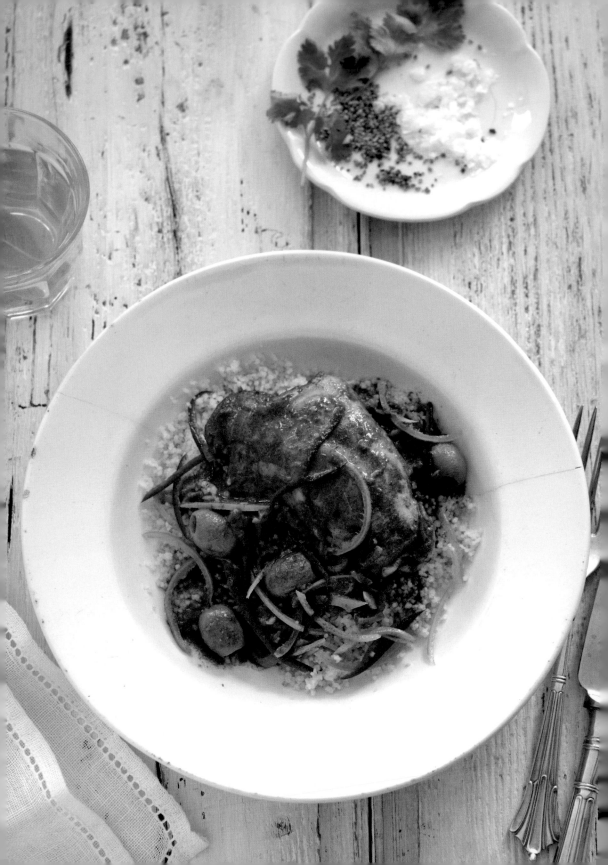

Chicken and Preserved Lemon Tagine

We all love this dish in my family. The only thing I have changed about it since my fat days is the amount of oil – I used to put in about 4 tablespoons – but nobody has ever noticed a difference!

Serves 4	7g FAT	1.3g SATURATES	3.3g SUGARS	1.19g SALT	215 CALORIES

1 tablespoon olive oil

1 large onion, peeled and finely chopped

2 teaspoons ground cumin

2 teaspoons ground coriander

2 teaspoons ground paprika

2 teaspoons ground cinnamon

2 teaspoons ground turmeric

3 garlic cloves, peeled and crushed

4 skinless chicken breasts or thighs

300ml chicken stock

a bunch of fresh coriander, roughly chopped

a handful of chopped fresh flat-leaf parsley

salt and freshly ground black pepper

10 green olives

rind of 1½ preserved lemons, cut into thin strips

1 red chilli (deseeded if preferred), finely sliced

Heat the oil in a large casserole and fry the onion really slowly until soft but not coloured. Add the spices and garlic and fry for a couple of minutes, stirring the whole time. If you have time, rub this mixture into the chicken thighs and pop them into the fridge to marinate for a few hours. If you don't have time, simply add the chicken to the pan and fry until the flesh becomes opaque – this should take a couple of minutes. Add the stock, half the coriander and the parsley. Season well, then cover and simmer over a really low heat for 10 minutes.

Meanwhile, put the olives into a small bowl and pour over enough boiling water to cover – this will remove the salty residue from the olives. Set aside for a few minutes, then drain.

Throw the strips of preserved lemon rind into the pan, stir in the olives and chilli and simmer until the meat is lovely and tender and cooked through. This will take about 20 minutes if you are using breasts, or 45 minutes if you are using thighs, but ensure that the meat is cooked through. Scatter over the remaining fresh coriander to serve.

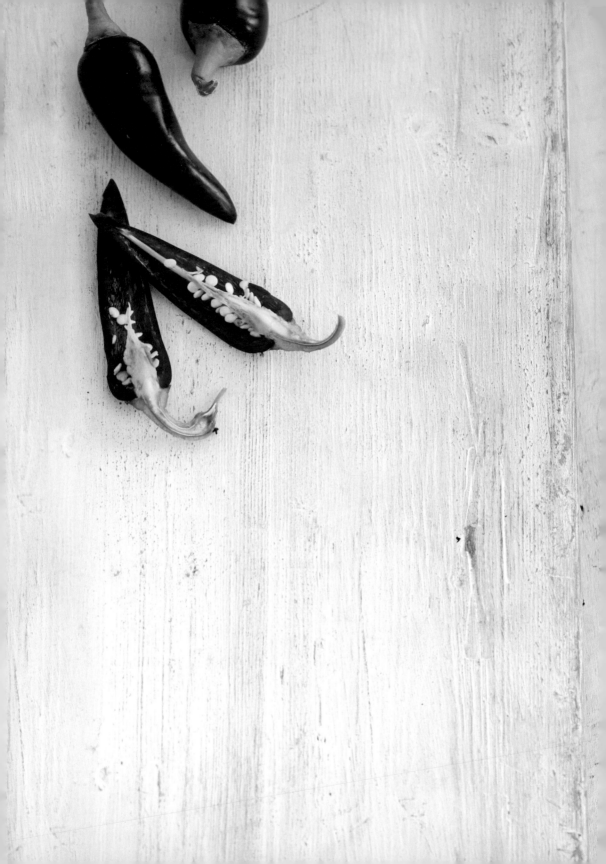

Delicious Dinner

'I always add a pile of vegetables or salad to whatever dish
I am making because I love to eat for as long as possible.
This is important – the act of eating is what we are often
drawn to. So eat for longer – just make sure it's something
green and healthy.'

Delicious Dinner

So, after the catastrophe of breakfast and the self-deceit of lunch, there, at the end of the day, looms... dinner.

Most of my life, the prospect of dinner offered up one of two things. It was either an opportunity to try to make good the trail of errors of the rest of the day, or it was my last chance of the day to truly reward myself. A little bit like the last obstacle in a steeplechase, this meal was a hurdle that, in my head, I could either soar over, or crash into! Generally, throughout my life, dinner has unfortunately been a case of the latter, the final domino to go over as I either binged myself in some weird rewarding system, or starved myself to undo the errors of lunch and breakfast.

I've always known I was in a terrible dilemma with my food whenever I tried to distinguish between dinner and that other odd sub-category of dining, supper. Usually, supper was just another prolonged excuse for having avoided dinner, OR it was the final, final hurrah – once I'd accepted the entire day had been a complete blowout. So, for me, throughout my life, dinner

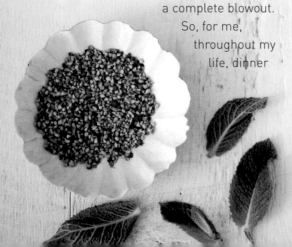

has been a curious culinary dance with the entire eating day that preceded it.

Dinner is invariably the one meal in the day when, as a sister, mother, wife or friend, I'm generally dining with other people and catering for a wide range of appetites. This is always dangerous because, when I'm cooking dinner for other people, it's easy to lose sight of my own appetite and my own needs. As a consequence, dinner is a mealtime that is all about weird acts of subterfuge, deceit, secret indulgence and, quite frankly, an awful lot of stress.

My husband has come up with a phrase to describe what I do when I'm in the midst of my weird relationship with eating, dieting and – dread of all dreads – BODY IMAGE. He calls it the 'Dinner Dodge'. He is, of course, referring to my approach to dinner when I've gorged myself on food for most of the day. Put simply, because I'm often cooking for my daughters, stepdaughters, parents and him, it's easy for me to be dovetailing between this and that dish as I try to cater for every single person's individual needs. Once all the fuss and nonsense of dining is done and the plates are empty, I realise I have got away with not serving myself a single morsel. As a result, as Mark would proclaim, I've managed to do the 'Dinner Dodge'. Not surprisingly, it's usually on the night of a dinner dodge that a suspect 'supper' decides to rear its ugly head!

The other rather clever (he insists it's clever!) phrase he's come up with for my approach to dinner is the Double D. No, not a reference to my rather ample (whatever weight I get down to) bra size, but more a description of the way in which I've managed to eat dinner twice. You know what it's like: you're frantically cooking everyone's food, you're worn out from a hard day's work and you simply can't help but pick, nibble, munch and dip as you go, often consuming hundreds of calories before anything even reaches the table. And then, to round things off brilliantly and bring the calories up to the thousands, you also sit down to eat dinner too. The Double D!

The new me, the me that loves food with a passion, but also loves feeling slimmer and healthier than I have in years, no longer plays the Dinner Dodge or indulges in the Double D. No! The new me knows very well that both of them lead to abject misery. So, I have various little tricks to ensure I stay 'safe' whenever I enter the very dangerous dinner zone:

- I always make myself a plate of healthy nibbles to chomp on while the girls have their tea. This means I no longer 'pick and nick' from their plates, leaving them starving and me fat!
- I never ever have a glass of wine on an empty stomach while cooking –

remember, it was invented by the Romans to open up the appetite – because, if I do, it always results in any resolve I may have built up going out the window. And I end up pie-eyed (literally!) and stuffed full of snacks.
- I always add a pile of vegetables or salad to whatever dish I am making because I love to eat for as long as possible! This is important - the act of eating is often what we are drawn to – so eat for longer, just make sure it is something green and healthy.
- If I'm having a particularly hungry day I will have a bowl of healthy soup before my meal to fill me up.
- I always have some carbohydrate at dinnertime. Otherwise, I end up feeling depraved – whoops, Freudian slip; of course, I meant to say deprived!
- I always drink water in a lovely crystal glass with 'ice-and-a-slice' in it whilst cooking in order to take the edge off my hunger. The pain of this abstemious behaviour is, of course, eased by the knowledge that I will almost certainly have a glass of wine with my dinner.
- I have done away with my 'hoover' style of eating and replaced it with the far more civilised, slow and considered chew! This way, I eat far less, and my stomach has time to tell my brain it's full, though Mark always does a cow impersonation when I eat.
- If I really want dessert, but know I have probably had enough calories for the day, I just have some cinnamon apples and low-cal ice cream, or a fruity ice lolly – that usually shuts me up!

Yummy Mummy

Sinless Spaghetti Bolognaise

I have yet to meet a man, woman or child who doesn't like spaghetti bolognaise, so it is an essential recipe for this book – just as it is for so many others. The difference with my recipe is that it's not loaded with calories, which means you can be greedy AND sinless!

Serves 4	7g FAT	1.9g SATURATES	11.8g SUGARS	0.76g SALT	378 CALORIES

1 tablespoon olive oil
1 onion, peeled and
   finely chopped
3 garlic cloves, peeled
   and crushed
2 celery sticks, finely chopped
2 carrots, peeled and
   finely chopped
400g minced turkey or lean
   minced beef
1 tablespoon tomato purée
2 x 400g cans chopped tomatoes
salt and freshly ground black
   pepper
200g mushrooms, chopped
2 bay leaves
200g wholewheat spaghetti
2 tablespoons freshly grated
   Parmesan cheese

Heat the olive oil in a large heavy-based pan and fry the onion and garlic over a low heat until soft but not coloured. Add the celery and carrots, reduce the heat and cook until soft.

Remove the veg from the pan, put in the minced turkey or beef and fry over a medium heat until lightly browned.

Return the vegetables to the pan, add the tomato purée and stir for about a minute. Pour in the tomatoes, bring up to the bubble, season with salt and pepper and stir in the chopped mushrooms and bay leaves. Reduce the heat and simmer gently for 30 minutes.

Meanwhile, cook the spaghetti according to packet instructions. Drain the spaghetti, toss it with the sauce and grate over the Parmesan.

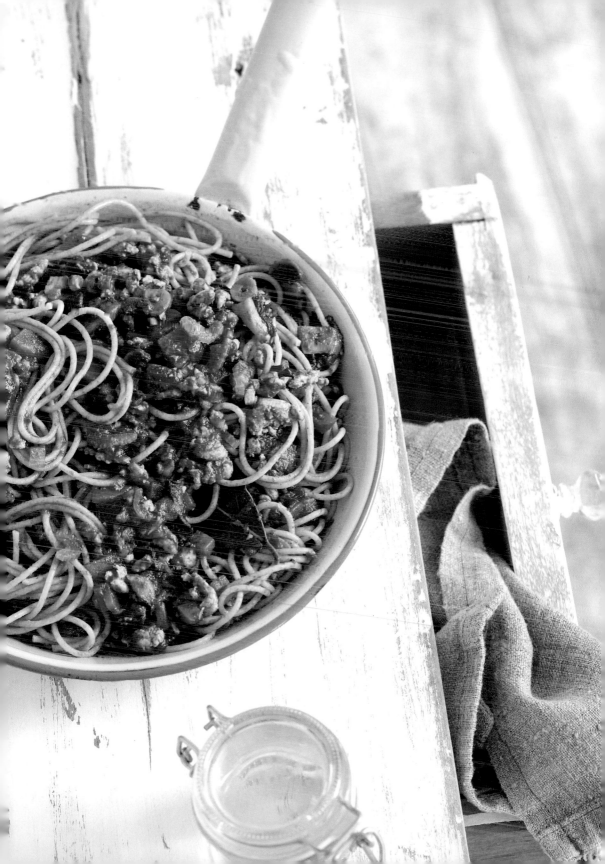

Lovely Ladies' Fingers

Okra is a massively underrated vegetable. Many people seem to find it boring – but that isn't the case with me. I simply love okra! It has a really subtle taste, but takes on and adopts other flavours really well. This dish goes beautifully with lamb, but is gorgeous on its own, too. Sometimes, for a treat, I have a little side dish of low-fat tzatziki alongside it.

Serves 4	7g FAT	0.6g SATURATES	11.5g SUGARS	1.51g SALT	153 CALORIES

750g small okra pods

olive oil spray

1 tablespoon sunflower oil

1 large onion, peeled and finely chopped

3 garlic cloves, peeled and left whole

1 tablespoon tomato purée

1 x 400g can tomatoes

2 teaspoons crushed coriander seeds

1 tablespoon Marigold vegetable bouillon powder (or a lamb stock cube)

salt and freshly ground black pepper

a squeeze of lemon juice (optional)

To garnish

1 teaspoon sunflower oil

1 teaspoon crushed coriander seeds

2 garlic cloves, peeled and finely chopped

Carefully remove the tops and tails of the okra, being careful not to cut in too far or they'll become slimy. Heat a wok until very hot, spray with olive oil spray, toss in the okra and fry for 4–5 minutes until they begin to brown all over; remove and set aside.

Reduce the heat, add 1 tablespoon sunflower oil and fry the onion and garlic cloves until really soft. Now add the tomato purée and fry until it begins to smell like fried tomato. Return the okra to the wok and tip in the tomatoes and crushed coriander seeds. Half-fill the empty tomato can with water, swish it around and pour the contents into the pan, along with the bouillon powder or crumbled stock cube. Season with freshly ground black pepper, cover with a lid and simmer over a very low heat for about 30 minutes or until the okra is tender. Check the seasoning; you may need to add a squeeze of lemon juice and a little salt.

For the garnish, heat the oil in a pan and fry the coriander seeds and garlic. Once you've dished up, sprinkle the garnish over the top.

Creamy Chicken Curry in a Hurry

This is one of the super-speedy dishes I fall back on all the time, because it's so easy to throw together and is also a real comfort food that the entire family loves. But it is strictly a family dish. I wouldn't serve it to guests – they might judge me slightly for its cheap thrills and tackiness. Thankfully, though, my family are stuck with me and they're not allowed any such judgements!

Serves 4   8g FAT | 2.1g SATURATES | 10.8g SUGARS | 0.95g SALT | 263 CALORIES

4 tablespoons korma curry paste

4 skinless chicken breasts, cut into 2cm chunks

150g low-fat Greek yogurt

400ml chicken stock

1 heaped tablespoon ground almonds

3 tablespoons sultanas

a small bunch of fresh coriander, chopped

First marinate the chicken. Dry-fry the korma paste in a frying pan until the aroma is released, tip into a bowl and set aside to cool. Stir 2 tablespoons of the yogurt into the korma paste, add the chicken pieces and give it all a good old mix. Set aside to marinate for as long as possible (you can leave it all day if you put it in the fridge).

When you are ready to cook, tip the chicken mixture into a frying pan. Pour over the stock, add the ground almonds and sultanas and bring to the boil. Reduce the heat to very low and simmer for 7–10 minutes. Turn off the heat, stir in the remaining yogurt, sprinkle over the coriander and serve with brown Basmati rice and salad. With this dish, I like a salad of thinly sliced lettuce, onions, red peppers and cucumber, dressed with nothing more than salt, a small squeeze of lemon juice and plenty of chopped fresh mint.

'Concentrate on conversation at the table rather than just hoovering up your food. Eat slowly, join in and chat.'

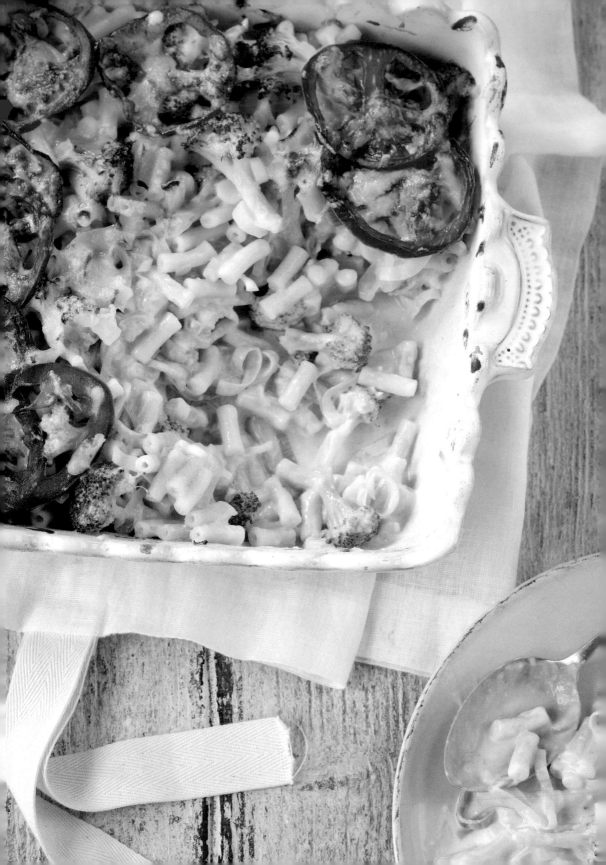

Marvellous Macaroni Cheese

My kids and I love macaroni cheese, as do most greedy girls! It does, however, have a rather annoying reputation for being fattening – although I have managed to shave off some of the calories by using skimmed milk and very strong cheese as, of course, the stronger the cheese, the less of the devilish stuff you need!

Serves 4	14g FAT	6.4g SATURATES	10.1g SUGARS	0.73g SALT	449 CALORIES

1 medium head of broccoli, cut into florets
250g macaroni
olive oil spray
1 leek, trimmed and finely sliced
25g light butter
2 tablespoons plain flour
2 teaspoons mustard powder
450ml warm skimmed milk
100g strong hard cheese, such as Parmesan cheese or extra mature Cheddar cheese
2 medium tomatoes, sliced

Steam the broccoli until just tender; drain under running cold water and set aside. Meanwhile, cook the macaroni according to packet instructions.

Spray a non-stick pan with oil and fry the leek until soft; remove from the pan and set aside. Melt the butter in the same pan, add the flour and cook, stirring constantly, for a minute. Add the mustard powder and carry on stirring while you gradually pour in the warmed milk. Keep stirring until the sauce thickens, then add three-quarters of the cheese (reserve some to sprinkle over the top). Preheat the grill to hot.

Drain the macaroni and stir it into the cheese sauce with the cooked broccoli and leeks. Pour the mixture into an ovenproof dish, arrange the sliced tomatoes around the edges of the dish and sprinkle over the remaining cheese. Pop under a hot grill until the cheese bubbles. This is lovely served with a crisp green salad.

Betty's Beautiful Burgers

I am very lucky to have my mum and dad as my next-door neighbours. Not only because I love them dearly, but also because my mum is a great cook and she always makes these for the girls when she is on babysitting duty!

Serves 4 (makes 8 burgers)

16g FAT | 6.6g SATURATES | 2.1g SUGARS | 0.56g SALT | 267 CALORIES

450g lean minced lamb
1 small onion, peeled and grated
1 garlic clove, peeled and grated
1 teaspoon tomato purée
2 teaspoons pomegranate
    molasses
zest of 1 unwaxed lemon and
    ½ tablespoon lemon juice
1 teaspoon ground cumin
2 teaspoons ground coriander
½ teaspoon ground cinnamon
5–6 tablespoons finely chopped
    fresh flat-leaf parsley (or
    2 tablespoons finely chopped
    fresh coriander)
2 tablespoons dried apricot
    stuffing, made up according
    to packet instructions (or
    use 1 egg, whisked, or 2
    tablespoons breadcrumbs
    bound with 1 egg)
vegetable oil, for brushing
salt and freshly ground black
    pepper

Put the lamb into a large mixing bowl, and add the onion, garlic, tomato purée, pomegranate molasses, lemon juice and zest, ground spices, chopped herbs and apricot stuffing (or egg/egg and breadcrumbs). Now prepare to get messy as you mix it up really well with your hands. Roll the mixture into 8 balls, each about the size of a clementine, and flatten each of them out between your hands into a patty about 1cm thick. Set aside in the fridge for a couple of hours to allow the flavours to mingle and the meat to firm up. About 15 minutes before you want to cook them, take the burgers out of the fridge.

Heat a heavy non-stick frying pan or griddle until very hot, then reduce the heat to medium. Brush a little oil onto the burgers, sprinkle them with some salt and black pepper and put them into the pan. Cook for 2–3 minutes on each side, taking care not to overcook them; it's better to have them slightly pink in the middle because they'll be nice and juicy. Put your burgers onto a warmed plate, cover them with kitchen foil and set aside to rest for a couple of minutes before serving. Serve with baked sweet potatoes and a tomato and onion salad.

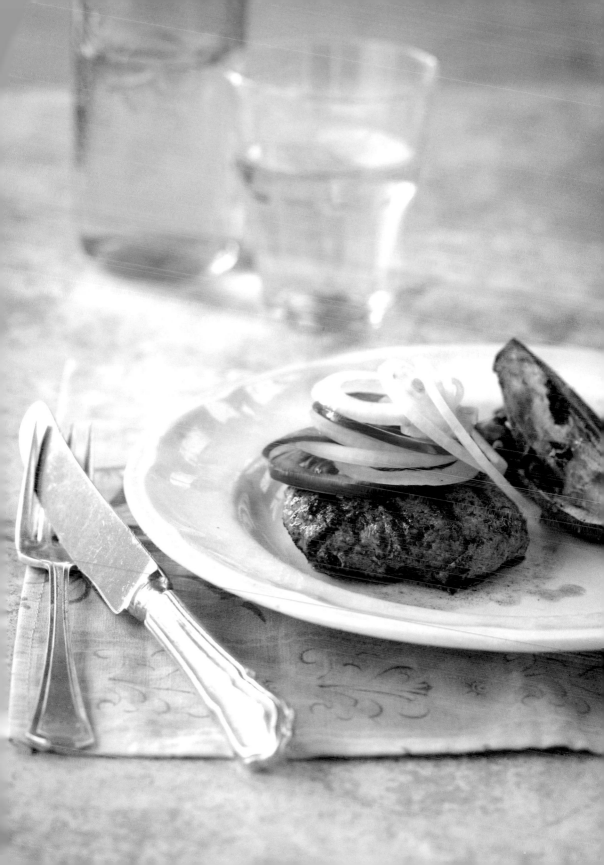

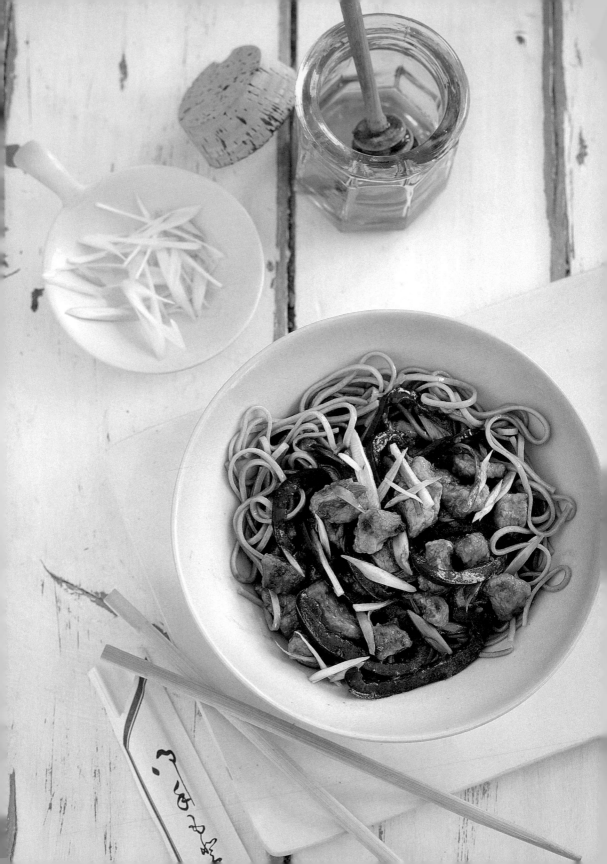

Sticky Honey Chinese Pork with Brown Rice Noodles

Fancy a Chinese? Well how about having one, but one that won't leave you feeling bloated and filled with regret? This recipe is light, tasty and filling – and just sweet enough – making it the perfect Chinese for you!

Serves 4	9g FAT	2.2g SATURATES	6.9g SUGARS	1.12g SALT	401 CALORIES

500g lean pork, cut into thin
   strips
1 tablespoon cornflour seasoned
   with salt and pepper
1 tablespoon runny honey
1 tablespoon soy sauce
1 tablespoon lemon juice
200ml chicken stock made from
   liquid concentrate
1 tablespoon vegetable oil
1 red pepper, thinly sliced
4 spring onions, finely sliced
1 teaspoon finely chopped garlic
1 teaspoon finely chopped fresh
   root ginger (optional)
200g brown rice noodles

Toss the pork in the cornflour, coating it evenly. Mix the honey, soy sauce, lemon juice and stock together in a bowl.

Heat the oil in a wok and cook the pork until it is just beginning to brown; set aside. Add the veg, garlic and ginger to the wok and cook for a few minutes, stirring the whole time. Throw the pork back into the pan and pour the honey mixture over it. Simmer until the pork is cooked through.

Meanwhile, prepare the brown rice noodles according to the packet instructions and serve.

My Big Sister's Pizza

My sister Dina is a fabulous cook, but like everyone else, she sometimes takes shortcuts in the kitchen. My girls love going to her house, as she is also super talented at art, too – so what could be better for any kids than painting while munching on pizza? Or indeed, painting their pizza with ingredients?! They always have strict instructions to bring me back a slice, or else I won't let them back in the house!

Serves 4	4g FAT	0.5g SATURATES	4.5g SUGARS	0.26g SALT	144 CALORIES

1 x 145g packet of pizza base mix
1 tablespoon olive oil
2 garlic cloves, peeled and
    finely chopped
500g small sweet tomatoes
handful of fresh basil leaves,
    torn, to garnish

Preheat the oven and prepare the pizza base dough according to the packet instructions. Roll it out fairly thinly and transfer it to a large baking tray.

Heat the olive oil in a non-stick saucepan and fry the garlic gently for 1–2 minutes until soft but not coloured. Add the tomatoes and simmer gently for 10 minutes over a low heat. Spread the sauce mixture over the pizza dough and bake in the oven according to packet instructions. To serve, scatter over plenty of torn basil leaves. How easy was that? Serve with a huge green salad to help fill you up!

'Run around like a maniac! Think of your metabolism as a fire that needs to be stoked with nourishing food and plenty of activity! I always charge up the stairs, hoover like crazy and chase my kids around until they squeal in delight and I work up a sweat!'

Thai Veggie Curry

This is a gorgeously creamy and fragrant curry that even the children will eat! I sometimes vary the recipe by adding extra chillies and lemongrass if I have some. You might like to try it with my Carrot and Mouli Salad (page 68).

Serves 4	14g FAT	6.9g SATURATES	17.4g SUGARS	1.37g SALT	248 CALORIES

1 tablespoon vegetable oil

1 medium onion, peeled and roughly chopped

4cm piece of fresh root ginger, peeled and finely chopped

2 large garlic cloves, peeled and crushed

70g Thai green curry paste

500g carrots, peeled and diagonally sliced into approx. 4cm lengths

500g courgettes, diagonally sliced into approx. 4cm lengths

1 tablespoon fish sauce

400g light coconut milk

200g fine green beans, sliced into 4cm lengths

a bunch of spring onions, diagonally sliced into 4cm lengths

4 handfuls of beansprouts

juice of 1 lime

2 tablespoons chopped fresh coriander

To serve
cooked brown rice, quinoa or rice noodles

Heat the oil in a large frying pan or wok and fry the onion, ginger and garlic until the onion is beginning to soften; don't allow it to colour.

Add the Thai curry paste to the pan or wok and stir for 1 minute. Stir in the carrots and courgettes, then add the fish sauce, coconut milk and 200ml water. Bring to the boil and simmer, uncovered, for 15 minutes.

Now add the green beans and spring onions and cook for a further 3 minutes, then throw in the beansprouts and cook for another couple of minutes. Squeeze over the lime juice and scatter over the chopped coriander. Serve with brown rice, quinoa or rice noodles

Chicken Shawarma

This is my all-time, most favourite street food ever – now there's a hard sell! It was always the first thing that we wanted to eat when we arrived in Amman, Jordan (my dad's home city) for our holidays. Of course, in those days, when I never thought about the size of my hips, I would always choose the fatty lamb variety. Nowadays I use the same recipe but just replace the lamb with far leaner chicken. If you ever eat another doner kebab after tasting one of these I will eat my hat (or rather I will eat your shawarma!). My favourite way to cook this is on the barbecue, but it does just as well under a grill.

Serves 4	15g FAT	2.4g SATURATES	0.8g SUGARS	1.5g SALT	293 CALORIES

For the shawarma

4 medium chicken breasts, cut into strips

2 tablespoons cider vinegar

juice of 1 lemon and 1 teaspoon grated lemon zest

1 teaspoon ground cinnamon

1 teaspoon ground allspice

1 teaspoon each of salt and freshly ground black pepper

½ teaspoon ground cardamom

3 pieces of mastic, finely ground

1 small onion, grated

1 small tomato, grated

3 slugs of olive oil

1 tablespoon finely chopped fresh flat-leaf parsley

For the tahini sauce

2 tablespoons tahini

1 tablespoon lemon juice

salt

2 tablespoons warm water

This is going to be so wonderfully simple you won't quite believe it! All you have to do is put all the shawarma ingredients in a bowl, stir really well, then set aside in the fridge to marinate for 24 hours. If you remember, it's nice to give it a stir every now and again.

To make the tahini sauce, put the tahini in a bowl, add the lemon juice with a good pinch of salt and slowly pour in the warm water, whisking all the time. Don't be frightened; the mixture might look sticky and horrible at first but, as you add more water (a little at a time), it will soon loosen up – you're after the consistency of single cream.

About an hour before you want to cook, take the chicken out of the fridge and strain it through a sieve. Arrange the chicken pieces on the barbecue (or on a grill tray if it's raining) and cook for a few minutes on each side until cooked through. To serve, pile the chicken into hot pitta breads, top with some salad and drizzle over the tahini sauce.

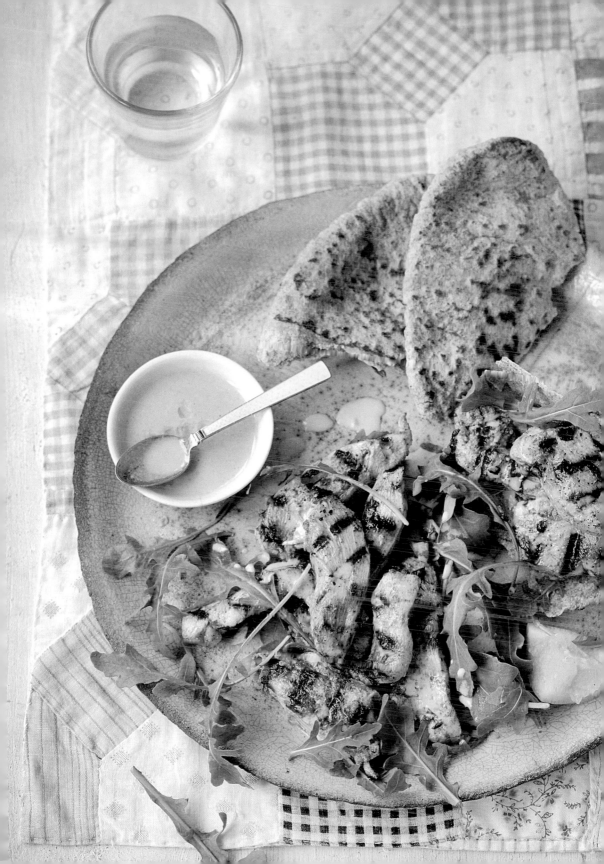

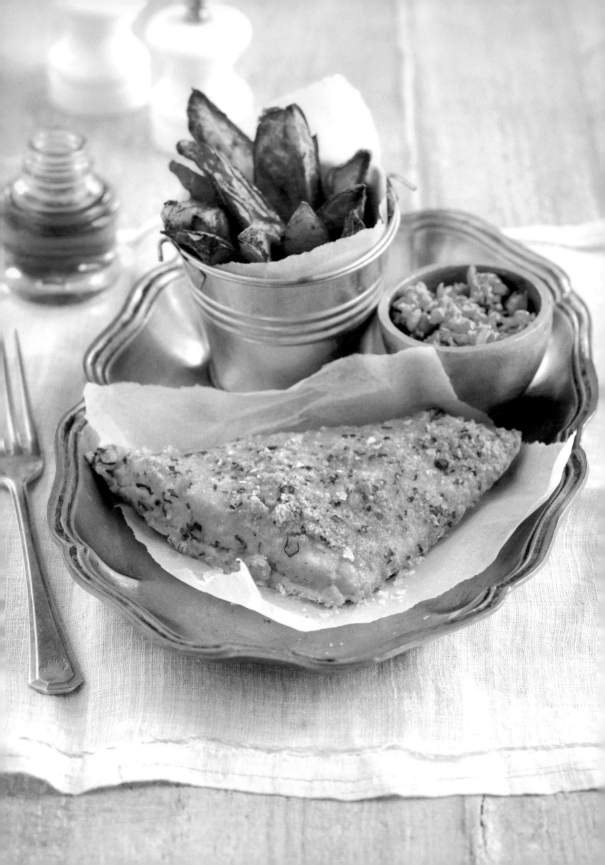

Funky Fish and Chips

This is our Friday night treat – what else can beat fish and chips on a Friday night other than fish and chips? Of course, you can make more chips for the rest of the family – but for all you greedy girls, stick to the amounts I've given.

Serves 4 | 4g FAT | 0.9g SATURATES | 2.1g SUGARS | 0.41g SALT | 367 CALORIES

4 x 200g haddock fillets

100g fine polenta

1 egg, beaten

10 fresh basil leaves, finely chopped

½ teaspoon chilli flakes

zest of ½ unwaxed lemon

a splash of milk

plain flour, for dusting

salt and freshly ground black pepper

For the chips

4 medium potatoes, peeled and cut into wedges

olive oil spray

salt and freshly ground black pepper

cayenne pepper

Preheat the oven to 200°C/gas mark 6. Put your potato wedges onto a large baking tray, spray with oil and season with salt, pepper and a light sprinkling of cayenne. Cook for about 20 minutes, at which point the fish will join them.

To make the coating for the fish, combine the polenta, egg, basil, chilli and lemon zest in a bowl and mix well. If necessary, you may need to add a splash of milk to give a fairly thick batter. Dust the fish with a little flour seasoned with salt and pepper, and dip it into the batter, ensuring it's thoroughly coated.

Pop the fish onto a baking tray and bake in the oven alongside the potatoes for about 20 minutes. Serve with mushy peas and good old-fashioned salt and vinegar.

Quinoa, Feta and Pomegranate Tabbouleh

This is my veggie sister's favourite ever salad. I love it too, but will often have a sneaky little grilled lamb chop (with fat removed, of course) on the side. You could, if you fancy, swap the feta cheese for grilled light halloumi and the pomegranate for watermelon – which also goes beautifully with mint.

Serves 4 | 20g FAT | 4.6g SATURATES | 13.4g SUGARS | 1.51g SALT | 468 CALORIES

300g quinoa
200g green beans, cut into 4cm lengths
a handful of sunflower seeds
200g low-fat feta cheese, crumbled
seeds from 1 pomegranate
2 tablespoons very finely chopped fresh mint leaves
2 tablespoons very finely chopped fresh flat-leaf parsley
4 medium tomatoes, deseeded and chopped into small pieces
4 spring onions, very finely chopped
3 tablespoons olive oil
3 tablespoons lemon juice
salt

Cook the quinoa according to packet instructions. Meanwhile, steam the beans until they are just beginning to soften; drain and refresh under cold running water. Dry-fry the sunflower seeds if you can be bothered – you don't have to, but they are much nicer that way.

Allow the quinoa, beans and seeds to cool down slightly (although this is nice served warm), then throw them into a salad bowl. Stir in the other ingredients and season with olive oil, lemon juice and a little salt – go easy on the salt because the feta itself is salty.

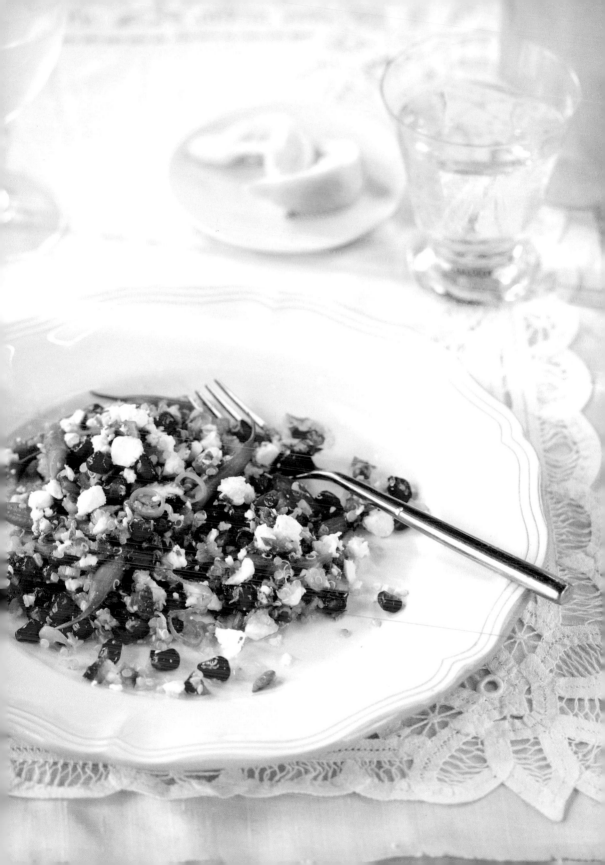

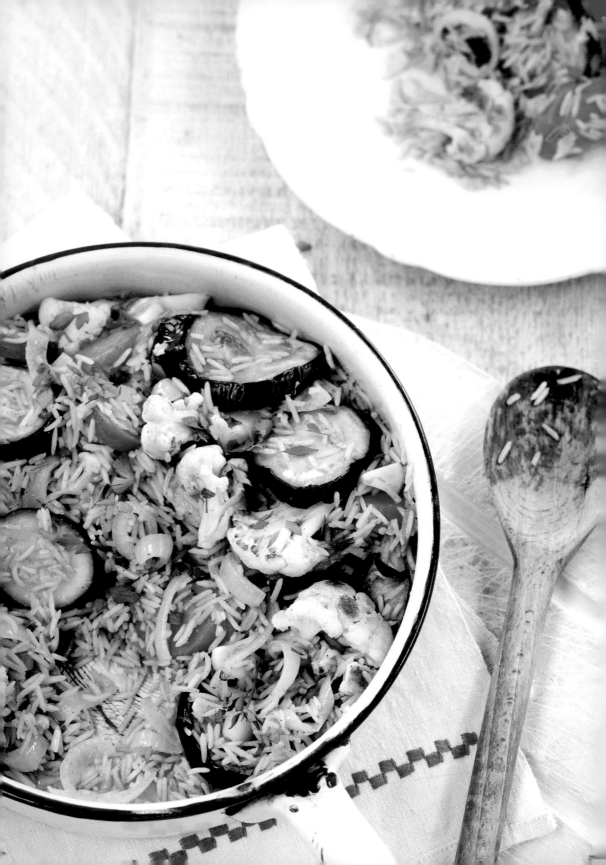

Vegetable Makloubeh

This is a real favourite childhood dish of mine. You can vary the vegetables according to taste and add broccoli if you like – just be sure to keep the same quantity of aubergine. Makloubeh means 'upside down', and this dish is usually made so that the rice is cooked on top of the veg and then the whole thing is turned out, but I have found it's very difficult to get everything evenly cooked this way, so created my own method. Sorry to any traditionalists out there!

Serves 4 | 8g FAT | 0.9g SATURATES | 14.7g SUGARS | 0.30g SALT | 333 CALORIES

1 medium aubergine, cut into 1.5cm-thick slices
spray olive oil
2 tablespoons olive oil
1 large onion, peeled and cut into 1cm-thick slices
2 large carrots, peeled and cut into 1cm-thick sticks
1 large courgette (or its equivalent in smaller ones), cut into 1cm-thick wedges
2 large garlic cloves, peeled and thickly sliced
salt and freshly ground black pepper
1 small cauliflower, broken into florets, plus any good leaves
180g white Basmati rice
½ teaspoon ground cinnamon
½ teaspoon ground allspice
500ml vegetable stock

Preheat the oven to 220°C/gas mark 7. Spray the aubergine pieces with olive oil and place on a flat baking tray. Roast for 10-15 minutes until they just begin to brown – keep an eye on them as you might need to turn them. Don't let them cook through at this stage, or they will disappear into the rice.

Meanwhile, heat the olive oil in a non-stick saucepan large enough to hold everything and gently fry the onion, carrots and courgettes until the onion begins to soften. Remove the vegetables with a slotted spoon and set aside. Mix in the sliced garlic, plenty of black pepper and a little salt.

Return the pan to the heat and add the cauliflower. Cover and fry until it begins to brown, shaking the pan. Remove and set aside with the other veg.

Tip the rice into the pan, add the spices and stir to release their aromas. Add the stock, bring to the boil and boil for 1 minute. Reduce the heat and simmer, covered, for 15 minutes. Stir in the vegetables, warm through and season. Keep an eye on the dish while it's cooking – if it looks too dry, add water, and if it looks too wet, take the lid off. Serve with a salad of tomatoes, cucumber and raw onion, dressed with salt, lemon and parsley.

Dinner Party Goddess

Prawn and Chorizo Rice Pot

I love chorizo, but the problem is that although it's incredibly tasty, it's also very fatty – so the answer is simply not to use very much. That way, you still get the great flavour without having to consume loads of calories. My husband hates chorizo, so I save this rather yummy dish for girls only nights! I know I bang on about using brown Basmati rice all the time, but with this dish I would throw caution to the wind and use white rice as I think it demands it.

Serves 4	7g FAT	2.8g SATURATES	4.9g SUGARS	1.16g SALT	367 CALORIES

70g chorizo
1 onion, peeled and
    finely chopped
3 garlic cloves, peeled and
    finely chopped
1 tablespoon smoked paprika
250g white Basmati rice
1 x 400g can tomatoes
350ml chicken stock made from
    liquid concentrate
salt and freshly ground black
    pepper
200g raw prawns

Dice the chorizo into tiny pieces and fry them in a large non-stick pan until they change colour. Add the onion and cook until soft. Stir in the garlic and paprika and cook for a further minute, stirring the whole time.

Now add the rice and pour in the tomatoes and stock. Bring up to the boil, stirring. Allow to bubble for a minute and season to taste – go easy on the salt because the stock will be salty already. Reduce the heat, cover and simmer for 10 minutes.

Stir in the prawns, replace the lid and cook for a further 5 minutes until the rice is tender.

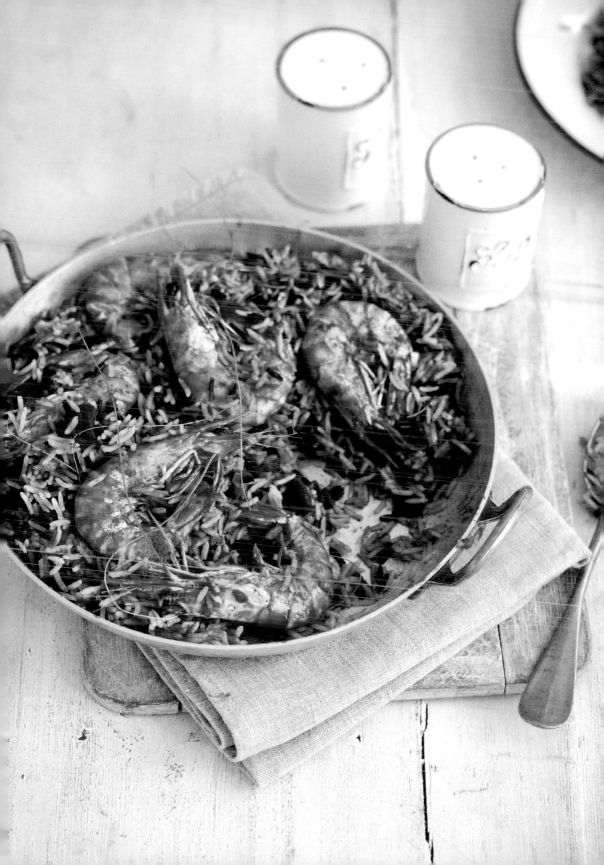

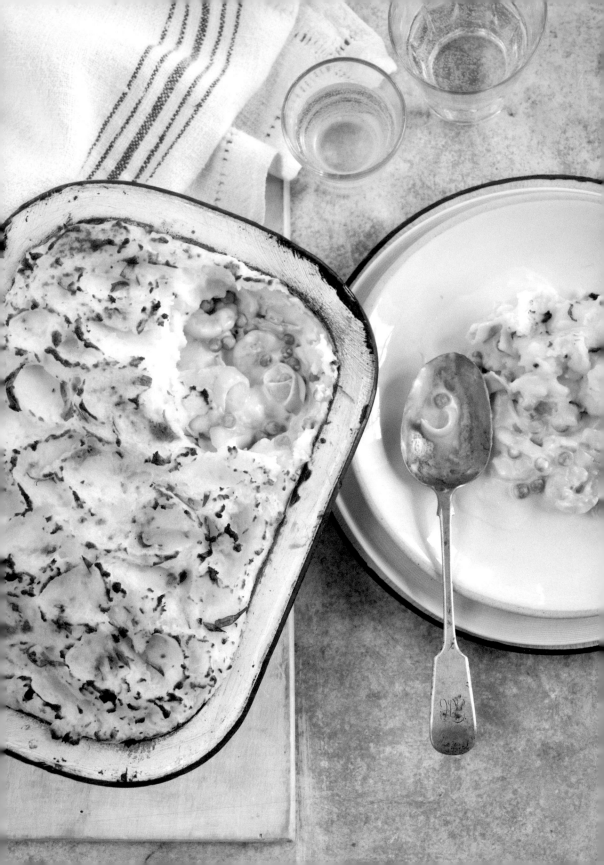

Fancy Fish Pie

This dish could easily be in the Yummy Mummy section because it's a great family meal. However, people always get excited when they see fish pie on the menu in a restaurant, so it's certainly good enough to serve at a dinner party.

Serves 4	9g FAT	3.6g SATURATES	10.4g SUGARS	2.72g SALT	451 CALORIES

500ml skimmed milk
½ onion, peeled and chopped
1 bay leaf
10 black peppercorns
300g boneless smoked haddock
300g coley fillets
12 raw peeled prawns
1 leek, trimmed and finely sliced
2 teaspoons light butter
120g natural very low-fat
    fromage frais
250g Philadelphia Extra Light
    cream cheese
a large handful of petits pois
1 tablespoon freshly grated
    Parmesan cheese

For the mash
800g potatoes, peeled and cut
    into chunks
salt and freshly ground black
    pepper
1 tablespoon light butter
a splash of milk
1 tablespoon chopped fresh
    tarragon

Boil the potatoes in salted water until tender. Drain, return to the pan and mash with the salt, pepper, butter and milk. Beat in the tarragon. Set aside.

Put the milk, onion, bayleaf and peppercorns into a large pan and heat gently until almost boiling. Reduce the heat to a very low simmer, gently lay in the haddock and coley pieces, cover with a lid and poach gently for 2 minutes. Add the prawns and continue to poach for a further minute until the fish flakes easily when poked with a fork. Using a slotted spoon, remove the fish. Skin and flake the fish, place in an ovenproof dish and cover with foil to keep warm. Strain the milk into a jug. Set aside.

In a medium non-stick pan, fry the leeks in the butter until soft but not coloured. Beat in the fromage frais and cream cheese, then whisk in 150ml of the reserved milk and the Parmesan

Cook the petits pois in boiling water and drain. Combine the peas with the fish in the ovenproof dish and pour the cream sauce over the top.

Preheat the grill to high. Carefully spoon the mashed potato over the top of the fish and scrape with a fork so you get lots of ridges that will crisp up nicely. Pop under the hot grill for 5 minutes until golden brown.

Fishy Business

This is a gorgeously light and summery dish – perfect to enjoy while sitting on a sunny patio with a glass of crisp white wine. A peppery rocket salad goes beautifully with it and gives it a little kick. I've used cod here, but you could use whatever white fish you like.

Serves 4	7g FAT	1g SATURATES	2.6g SUGARS	0.41g SALT	222 CALORIES

400g baby new potatoes

120g petits pois

2 tablespoons olive oil

juice and zest of ½ unwaxed lemon

1 tablespoon capers

1 tablespoon chopped fresh flat-leaf parsley

salt and freshly ground black pepper

sunflower oil spray

4 x 100–150g chunky cod fillets (or use another white fish)

Scrub the potatoes and cook in boiling salted water until tender, adding the petits pois for the last few minutes. Drain, return to the pan and roughly crush together using a fork.

In a small bowl, mix together the oil, lemon juice and zest, capers, parsley and seasoning.

Spray a non-stick frying pan with oil. Dry the fish with kitchen paper and fry in the pan for about 3 minutes on each side or until cooked through. To serve, lay the fish on top of the crushed potato and peas, then drizzle the dressing on top.

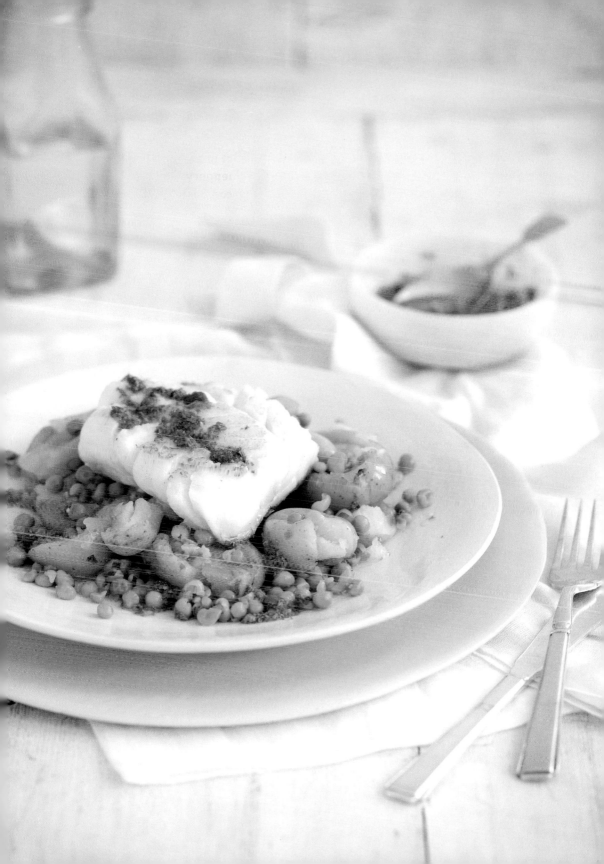

Chilli con Carne

This is one of those dishes that tastes even better the next day, so I'll often make a big batch on a Sunday if I know I've got a busy week ahead. Try it with a jacket potato one night and rice the next. Variety is, after all, the spice of life!

Serves 4	20g FAT	6.3g SATURATES	11.3g SUGARS	1.19g SALT	534 CALORIES

450g lean minced beef
½ tablespoon olive oil
1 large onion, peeled and sliced
1 green pepper, sliced
3 garlic cloves, peeled and
    crushed
1 small red chilli (deseeded if
    preferred), finely chopped
1 teaspoon each of cumin and
    coriander seeds, ground
1 x 400g can tomatoes
250ml beef stock made from
    liquid concentrate
1 tablespoon tomato purée
1 x 200g can kidney beans
2 bay leaves
200g brown rice

For the salsa
1 small avocado, peeled and
    finely diced
2 ripe tomatoes, finely diced
¼ cucumber, finely diced
2 tablespoons finely chopped
    red onion
salt
a good squeeze of lemon juice
small handful of chopped fresh
    coriander

Heat a large non-stick saucepan and dry-fry the beef until browned. Remove from the pan and set aside on a plate. Heat the oil in the same pan and fry the onion, green pepper and garlic until soft. Add the chilli and spices and fry for a further minute, stirring the whole time. Cover the pan with a lid and let everything cook down for 5–7 minutes over a very low heat.

Pour in the tomatoes and beef stock, increase the heat and stir in the tomato purée, kidney beans and beef. Tuck the bay leaves into the sauce. Bring the whole thing up to the boil, then reduce the heat and simmer for 30–40 minutes – you may need to add more water if it looks like it's drying out.

Meanwhile, cook the rice according to packet instructions and prepare the salsa by mixing together all the ingredients in a little bowl.

To serve, divide the rice between 4 bowls, pile the chilli on top and accompany with the salsa.

Herby Veal Stew

This recipe would work just as well with pork or chicken, and you could also swap the herbs for any others you fancy. Serve with a small portion of herby mash or some steamed new potatoes and steamed cabbage or green beans.

Serves 4   11g FAT | 3.6g SATURATES | 8.7g SUGARS | 0.55g SALT | 335 CALORIES

1½ tablespoons olive oil

800g diced stewing veal

2 carrots, peeled and sliced

2 medium onions, peeled and sliced

3 good-sized sprigs of fresh lovage

150ml dry white wine

150ml chicken stock

salt and freshly ground black pepper

1 tablespoon cornflour mixed with 2 tablespoons cold water

3 tablespoons chopped fresh chervil (optional)

Heat the oil in a large casserole and brown the meat in small batches over a high heat; remove from the pan and set aside on a plate. Add the carrot and onion to the same pan, reduce the heat to medium, and fry for about 5 minutes until the onion begins to colour.

Return the meat to the pan and drop in the lovage. Warm the wine and stock and pour over the meat. Season well, taking into account the saltiness of the stock, and bring to the boil. Reduce the heat to a very slow simmer, cover with a lid and cook for 1½ hours until the meat is tender.

Remove the meat and vegetables from the pan with a slotted spoon. Whisk the cornflour mixture into the remaining liquid and bring to the boil; simmer for 2–3 minutes until the sauce thickens. Return the meat and vegetables to the pan and adjust the seasoning if necessary. If you are using the chervil, add it to the stew just before serving.

'Remember, don't drink on an empty stomach – wine opens up the appetite. Have a glass of sparkling water instead, and save your glass of wine for when you eat.'

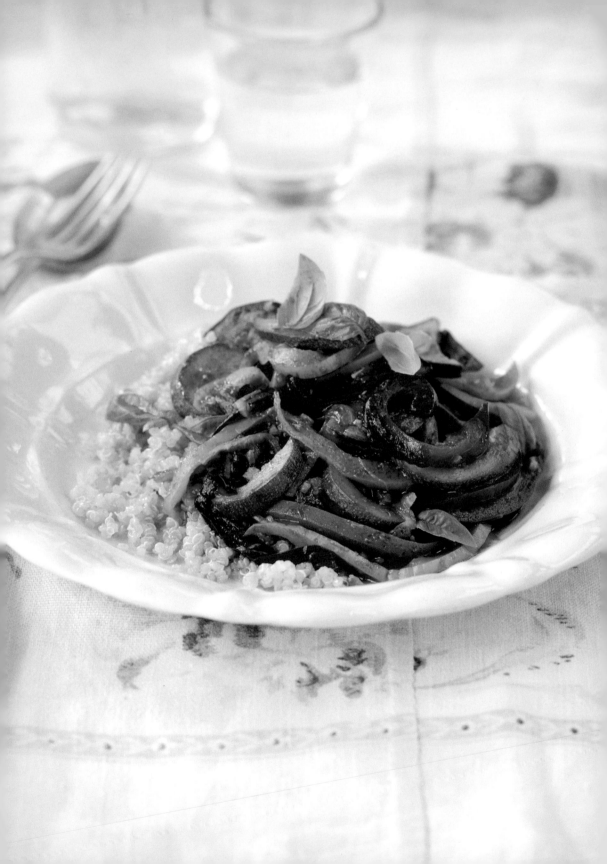

Ratatouille with Quinoa

What you're getting with this dish is a real taste of the summer. To get the best from a ratatouille, don't make the mistake of cooking and boiling everything together so that it becomes a garbled mush of general vegetable flavour. The art of ratatouille is to treat each ingredient with the respect it deserves – and if you do that, it will be delicious. The joy of a good ratatouille is not only how gorgeous it tastes, but also how gorgeous it looks.

Serves 4 | 10g FAT | 1g SATURATES | 19.1g SUGARS | 0.15g SALT | 319 CALORIES

1 medium aubergine, cut into rough cubes
olive oil spray
salt and freshly ground black pepper
2 tablespoons olive oil
2 onions, peeled and sliced
5 garlic cloves, peeled and roughly chopped
1 red pepper, sliced
1 yellow pepper, sliced
1 green pepper, sliced
4 courgettes, chopped into chunks
1 x 400g can tomatoes (use the best quality possible)
1 tablespoon tomato purée
200g quinoa
a handful of torn fresh basil leaves

Preheat the oven to 180°C/gas mark 4. Lightly spray the aubergine cubes with oil, spread them out on a baking tray and sprinkle with salt. Roast for 15–25 minutes, until golden brown.

Meanwhile, heat the oil in a large ovenproof casserole and fry the onion and garlic until soft but not coloured. Lay the sliced peppers on top and put on a tight-fitting lid. Reduce the heat and simmer very gently for 10 minutes until the peppers start to soften. Add the courgettes, tomatoes and tomato purée, season with salt and pepper and bring to the boil. Tip in the roasted aubergines, then transfer the casserole to the oven and cook for 40 minutes.

While the ratatouille is cooking, steam the quinoa according to packet instructions. To serve, scatter the basil leaves over the ratatouille and accompany with the steamed quinoa.

Winey Chicken

This is my answer to the classic coq au vin! It's a definite crowd pleaser and is one of those dishes that mothers and mother-in-laws absolutely adore. Petits pois and baby new potatoes are a fabulous addition. Just watch out that the mothers and mother-in-laws don't end up taking the 'winey' side of this dish any further than the chicken. My stepdaughters laugh at the name of this dish – because it makes them think of a chicken whining!

Serves 4	5g FAT	1.4g SATURATES	4.4g SUGARS	0.62g SALT	211 CALORIES

½ tablespoon olive oil

1 medium onion, peeled and very finely chopped

a handful of button mushrooms, kept whole or halved

2 teaspoons tomato purée

a small glass of white wine (I said 'small'!)

250ml chicken stock made from liquid concentrate

4 chicken thighs (or breasts), skin removed, either left whole or sliced

1 teaspoon cornflour mixed with a little cold water

4 tablespoons finely chopped fresh flat-leaf parsley, to garnish

For the pretty croûtons
3 slices of brown bread
olive oil spray

Heat the oil in a non-stick casserole and fry the onion really slowly until soft but not coloured. If the oil doesn't seem to be enough, splash a little chicken stock in, too. Throw in the mushrooms and cook for a few minutes, stirring all the time. Now add the tomato purée and, still stirring, fry for 30 seconds. Pour in the wine and bring up to the bubble, then add the stock and the chicken. Simmer over a really low heat for about 25–35 minutes until cooked through. (If you are using breasts, they will take less time, approx. 15–20 minutes, and even less if sliced.)

While the chicken is cooking, make the pretty croûtons. Using a cookie cutter, cut the bread into little heart shapes. Spray with oil and fry in a hot non-stick frying pan until golden brown; set aside.

When the chicken is cooked through, take it out of the sauce and set aside on a plate while you thicken the sauce. Whisk the cornflour mixture into the pan and simmer until the sauce thickens. To serve, put the chicken back into the sauce, sprinkle with the parsley and adorn with your beautiful heart-shaped croûtons. Serve with baby new potatoes and petits pois.

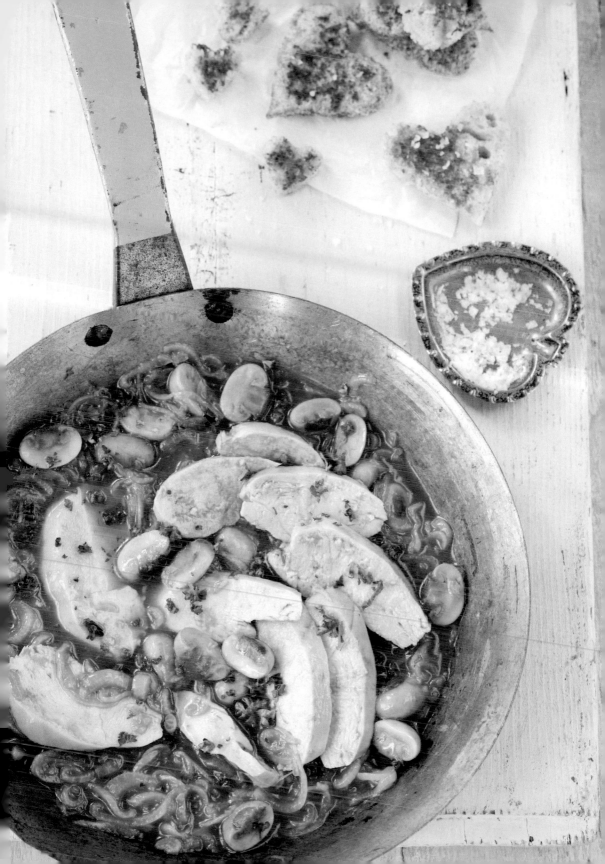

Fabulous Falafels

I always make these falafels if I'm having vegetarians over on the same night as I'm cooking Shawarma (page 116) for my non-veggie friends. I think they are the best two street-food dishes ever – easy to make, super cheap and utterly delicious. My Carrot Salad (page 76) goes really well with this dish.

Serves 4	4g FAT	0.8g SATURATES	3.8g SUGARS	3.09g SALT	245 CALORIES

1 x 400g can chick peas, drained
1 teaspoon salt
1 teaspoon ground cumin
1 teaspoon ground coriander
1 teaspoon cayenne pepper
1 large garlic clove, peeled
   and crushed
zest of ½ unwaxed lemon
1 teaspoon bicarbonate of soda
1 tablespoon very finely chopped
   fresh coriander
vegetable oil spray
4 warmed wholemeal pitta
   breads

For the dressing
150g low-fat Greek yogurt
1 small garlic clove, peeled
   and crushed
100g chopped rocket

Preheat the oven to 220°C/gas mark 7. Put the chick peas, salt, spices, garlic, lemon zest, bicarbonate of soda and chopped coriander into a food processor and lightly blend to a coarse purée. Wet your hands to stop the mixture sticking to them and shape the mixture into 16 patties. Spray a baking tray with oil, arrange your falafels on top and lightly spray them all over with a fine mist of oil. Bake for 15–20 minutes, turning once.

While the falafels are cooking, make the dressing by beating together the yogurt with the crushed garlic and rocket in a bowl. If necessary, you may need to thin the mixture with a couple of tablespoons warm water to a coating consistency. Serve the falafels inside the warmed pitta breads and top with the yogurt dressing.

Saffron Prawns with Rice

This glorious dish, fragrant with saffron, ginger and garlic, is a perfect supper to share with friends. If you have some fresh coriander you could add a flourish at the end for a bit of extra colour and perfume.

Serves 4   4g FAT | 0.6g SATURATES | 1g SUGARS | 1.83g SALT | 292 CALORIES

1 tablespoon olive oil

450g raw peeled prawns

olive oil spray

2 large garlic cloves, peeled
  and crushed

¼ teaspoon ground saffron (or
  5–6 saffron strands soaked in
  1 tablespoon boiling water)

1 teaspoon grated fresh root
  ginger

¼ teaspoon cayenne pepper
  (optional)

180g Basmati rice

zest of 1 unwaxed lemon

2 tablespoons frozen peas

1 teaspoon salt

a bunch of spring onions, finely
  chopped

Heat the oil in a large heavy-based saucepan and fry the prawns over a high heat until they turn pink all over. Remove from the pan and set aside on kitchen paper.

Lightly spray the same pan with oil and put in the garlic, saffron, ginger and cayenne. Stir-fry for 1–2 minutes so the spices release their aromas, and then add the rice, lemon zest and peas. Pour over enough water to cover the rice by about 1.5cm and bring to the boil, stirring. Cover with a lid and simmer for 15 minutes or until most of the water has been absorbed.

Stir in the prawns, salt and spring onions and serve immediately with a huge green salad containing lots of fresh herbs.

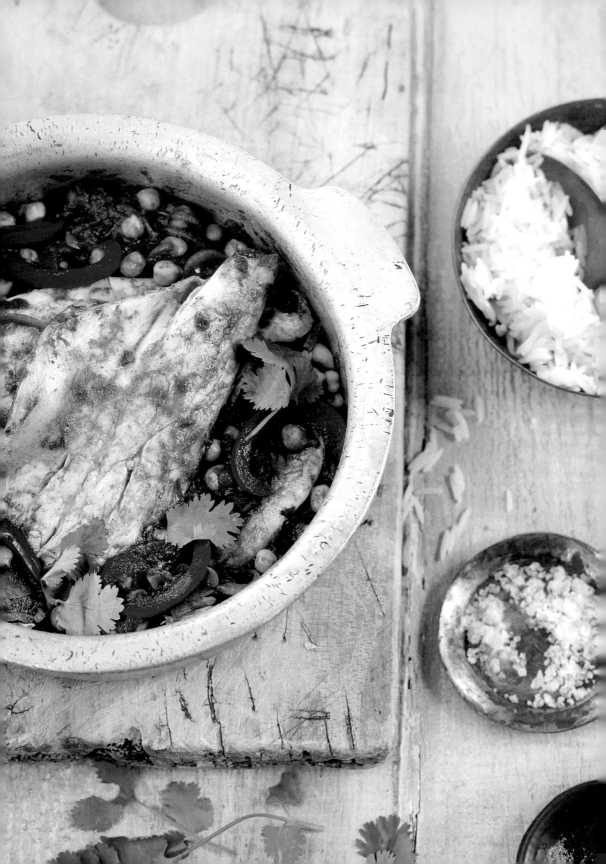

Moroccan-Style Fish

I will admit, fish is not my favourite food and my Dad feels just the same. We reckon it's because my father was a Bedouin and you don't find many fish in the desert! It just doesn't feel right, quite apart from the fact that I'm always left feeling a bit hungry at the end of a fish meal – especially if it hasn't had a pile of chips plonked alongside it. So, I invented this recipe especially for me and my Dad. It has loads of gorgeous spices, rich tomatoes and herbs. It really is delicious and I always serve it with a couple of spoonfuls of rice, not only to mop up the delicious juices, but also to ease the pain of not having any chips.

| Serves 4 | 7g FAT | 0.9g SATURATES | 7.8g SUGARS | 0.61g SALT | 409 CALORIES |

1 tablespoon olive oil
1 onion, peeled and thinly sliced
1 red pepper, cut into strips
3 garlic cloves, peeled and
   quartered
2 tablespoons ground paprika
2 teaspoons ground cumin
1 x 400g can tomatoes
zest of 1 unwaxed lemon
1 x 400g can chick peas, drained
salt and freshly ground black
   pepper
4 x 100g white fish fillets, such
   as cod or coley (you could also
   use snapper, although it isn't
   white)
a large handful of fresh
   coriander, chopped
200g brown rice

Preheat the oven to 160°C/gas mark 3. Heat the oil in a large casserole and fry the onion and pepper until soft. Add the garlic and spices and stir them around until their aromas are released. Stir in the tomatoes and lemon zest, bring up to the bubble, then reduce the heat and simmer for 15 minutes.

Add the chick peas and simmer for a further 5 minutes. Season with salt and pepper, put the fish on top and transfer to the oven for 20 minutes, covering with a lid or foil.

Meanwhile, prepare the rice according to packet instructions. When the fish is ready, sprinkle with chopped coriander and serve with brown rice.

Roasted Red Peppers with Feta

This is a super-duper easy dish that you can make more substantial by serving with rice or potatoes and some extra green veg or salad. Stuffed peppers also make a great side dish for serving alongside roast lamb, pork or fish.

Serves 4	17g FAT	6g SATURATES	21.3g SUGARS	2.26g SALT	313 CALORIES

8 red peppers
salt and freshly ground black
    pepper
32 cherry tomatoes
300g light feta cheese, cut
    into cubes
8 teaspoons olive oil
olive oil spray
a handful of garlic cloves, left
    whole and unpeeled
a couple of handfuls of fresh
    basil leaves, to garnish

Preheat the oven to 200°C/gas mark 6. Slice the tops off the peppers, keeping their stalks intact, and set aside. Scoop out the seeds and the white pith and season the insides with salt and pepper. Stuff the peppers with the tomatoes and a few chunks of the feta and season with a little black pepper. Drizzle 1 teaspoon olive oil into each pepper.

Spray a baking tray that is just large enough to hold the peppers with a little olive oil. Stand the peppers upright inside the dish and scatter the garlic cloves on to the tray. Put the lids on the peppers and bake for about 45 minutes until the peppers and tomatoes are soft. Garnish with the basil leaves and serve with the roasted garlic cloves.

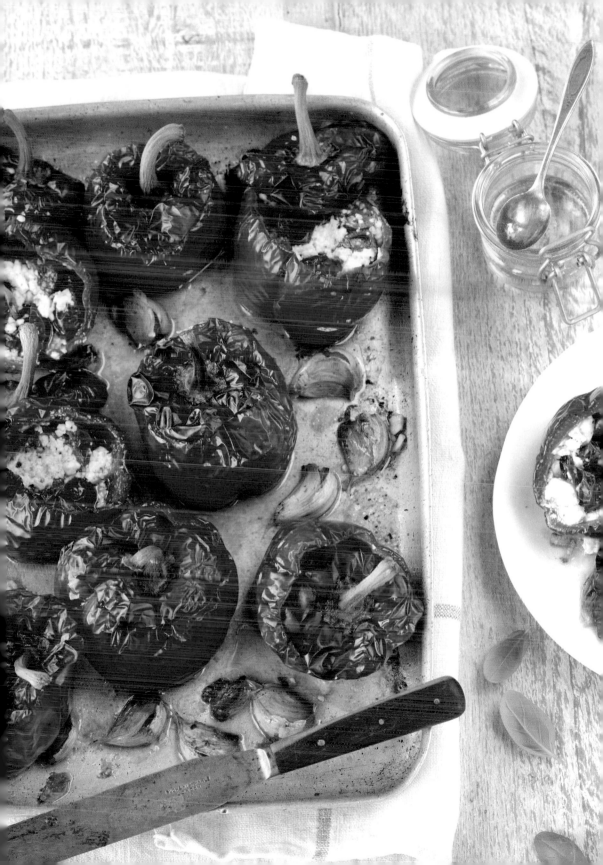

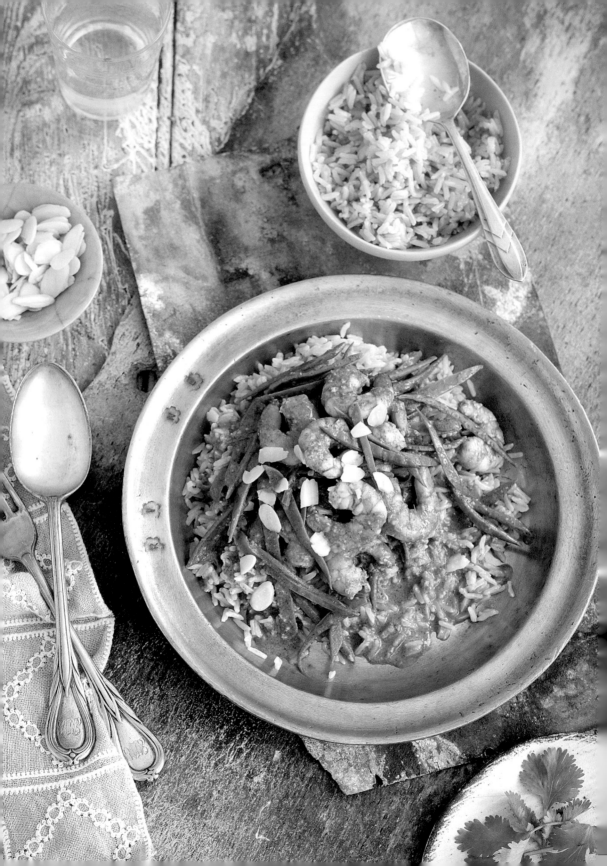

Dinner for Two

Coconut, Prawn and Mangetout Curry

This is always my husband's favourite dish whenever we order a takeaway. Traditionally, I would always look on in horror – and envy – as he poured it all out and proceeded to tuck into God knows how many calories! This version, which I've now converted him to, is only half as bad for you, simply through the use of light coconut milk, which still has all the flavour but half the fat. The only deal me and my hubby have now is that when I serve it up to him I have to pop it in a tin foil box, and then into a plastic bag before going outside and knocking on the door!

Serves 2 27g FAT | 12.3g SATURATES | 4.9g SUGARS | 1.88g SALT | 406 CALORIES

1 tablespoon vegetable oil
1 garlic clove, peeled and
  finely chopped
2 tablespoons Madras curry
  paste
300ml light coconut milk
1 tablespoon ground almonds
300g raw peeled king prawns
75g mangetout
1 tablespoon brinjal (aubergine)
  pickle
a handful of chopped fresh
  coriander, to garnish

Heat the oil in a frying pan, add the garlic and fry until soft. Stir in the curry paste and cook for 1 minute, stirring the whole time. Pour in the coconut milk, add the ground almonds and simmer gently for 10 minutes.

Throw in the prawns and cook very gently until they turn pink (don't overcook them or they will be tough). Add the mangetout and continue to simmer gently for a few more minutes. Finally, stir in the brinjal pickle. Garnish with the coriander. Serve with steamed brown rice.

Lemony Risotto

This wonderfully fragrant dish is a perfect reminder of mine and Mark's honeymoon on the Amalfi Coast in Italy. Needless to say, when we ate it back then it was rapidly followed by a bottle or two of limoncello and then a cracking hangover. The version we ate was also rounded off with an enormous knob of butter, while this one avoids that last flurry of indulgence. Risotto is all about getting into the stirring vibe – and the creamy, dreamy texture is perfect for a romantic night in!

Serves 2	10g FAT	2.5g SATURATES	5.9g SUGARS	1.02g SALT	463 CALORIES

200g asparagus, trimmed

80g petits pois

1 tablespoon finely chopped
   fresh mint

grated zest of 1 unwaxed lemon

a handful of fresh basil

salt and freshly ground black
   pepper

1 tablespoon olive oil

4 spring onions, sliced into
   2cm lengths

1 garlic clove, peeled and
   finely chopped

150g Arborio risotto rice

100ml dry white wine

800ml hot chicken or vegetable
   stock

2 tablespoons freshly grated
   Parmesan cheese

a handful of watercress

Steam the asparagus until tender and set aside. Cover the peas in boiling water, leave for a few minutes, then drain and set aside. In a small bowl, mix together the mint, lemon zest, basil and some seasoning; set aside.

Heat the oil in a large non-stick saucepan and fry the spring onions and garlic until soft but not coloured. Add the rice and stir for a minute, then add the wine and keep stirring until all the wine has been absorbed. Gradually add the hot stock, a ladleful at a time, keeping the liquid on a simmer and ensuring that each ladleful has been absorbed before you add the next. Stir continuously until you have used up all the stock, by which time the rice should be soft. If it isn't cooked, just add a bit more stock and carry on stirring for a bit longer.

Finally stir in the steamed vegetables and the herb-and-lemon mixture. To serve, divide the risotto between 2 bowls, scatter over the Parmesan and top with a little mound of watercress.

Spicy Lamb Chops

I love anything thrown on the barbecue, but lamb on the barbie really is quite sublime. My husband, on the other hand, doesn't like barbies or lamb, so it was a real act of love when he enlisted my mum's help last summer to surprise me with this romantic meal. Ahhhh, the way to this woman's heart is definitely through the stomach!

Serves 2   13g FAT | 6g SATURATES | 4.7g SUGARS | 0.2g SALT | 245 CALORIES

---

1 teaspoon ground cumin

zest of 1 unwaxed lemon

juice of ½ lemon

½ tablespoon pomegranate
    molasses

3 sprigs of fresh rosemary,
    finely chopped

1 garlic clove, peeled
    and crushed

4 French trimmed lamb cutlets

1 medium aubergine, sliced

olive oil spray

2 tablespoons pomegranate
    seeds, to garnish

To make the marinade for the lamb, combine the cumin, lemon zest and juice, pomegranate molasses, rosemary and garlic in a bowl. Rub the mixture into the lamb cutlets and set aside to marinate in the fridge for a few hours.

To cook the lamb, grill or barbecue for 3–7 minutes on each side, depending on how you like it cooked.

Spray the aubergine slices with olive oil and grill at the same time as the lamb until soft on the inside and golden brown on the outside.

Transfer the lamb to a plate and set aside to rest for 5 minutes so it's nice and tender. To serve, pile the aubergines onto 2 plates, top with the lamb cutlets and scatter over the pomegranate seeds. Serve with hummus and my Carrot Salad (page 76).

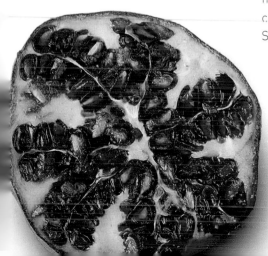

Shredded Duck, Watercress and Pomegranate Salad

Quack, quack! Traditionally, duck is not something you would expect to find on the menu of anyone who is watching their weight. BUT, like pork, if you get rid of the skin and the fat, duck is, in fact, quite a lean meat. So, put it back in your shopping basket next time you're in the supermarket. This duck salad is probably one of the lightest, brightest ways to enjoy a balmy summer evening with a loved one...

Serves 2	3.6g FAT	0.5g SATURATES	16.9g SUGARS	3.89g SALT	299 CALORIES

2 duck breasts
1 teaspoon five spice powder
4 tablespoons rice wine vinegar
4 tablespoons reduced salt
   soy sauce
5 tablespoons pomegranate juice
200g watercress
140g chicory leaves
seeds of 1 large pomegranate

Preheat the oven to 200°C/gas mark 6. Skin the duck breasts, dry them with kitchen paper and rub the flesh all over with five spice powder.

Combine the vinegar, soy sauce and pomegranate juice in a small roasting tin and put in the duck breasts. Cover with foil and bake for 40 minutes. Remove from the oven and set aside on a plate to cool down. Meanwhile, pour off any fat from the pan and allow the cooking juices to cool down.

Once the meat is cool enough to handle, shred the flesh using 2 forks. Scatter the watercress, chicory and pomegranate seeds over 2 plates, add the shredded duck meat and drizzle over the warm cooking juices to serve.

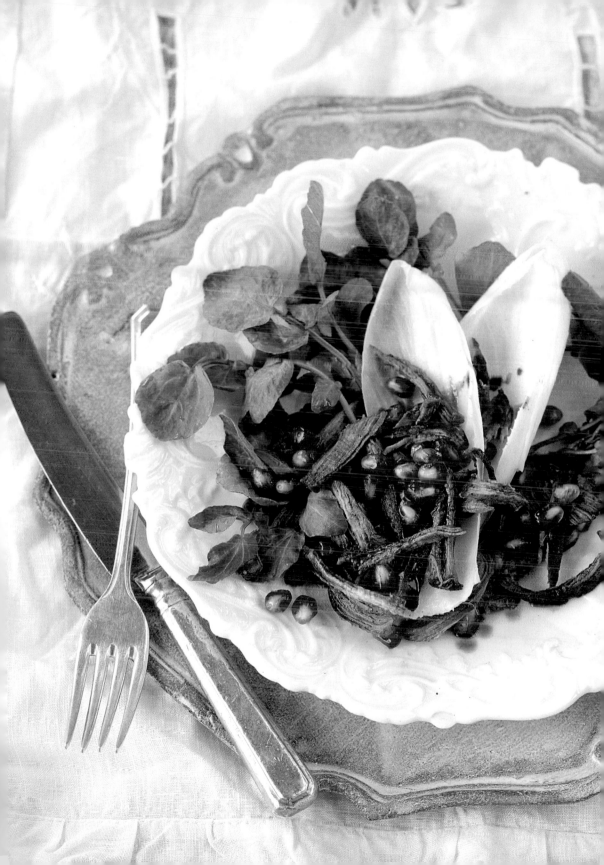

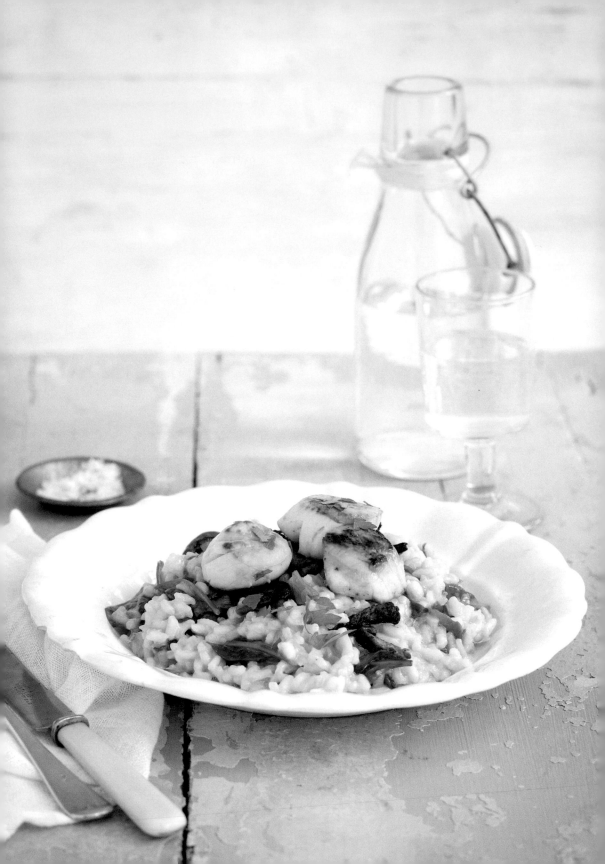

Risotto with Seared Scallops

This is definitely a show-offy dish designed to 'pull' and impress. Oh yes, remember, pop a glass of champagne alongside the plate!

Serves 2	14g FAT	3g SATURATES	3.4g SUGARS	1.97g SALT	551 CALORIES

For the risotto
1 tablespoon olive oil
1 small onion, peeled and
    finely chopped
175g Arborio risotto rice
50ml dry white wine
650ml warm chicken stock
150g baby leaf spinach
zest of ½ unwaxed lemon
25g light butter
salt and freshly ground black
    pepper

For the scallops
1 teaspoon olive oil
2 rashers of back bacon with all
    visible fat removed
4 fresh sea scallops, rinsed and
    patted dry
1 tablespoon dry white wine (or
    use chicken stock)

1 tablespoon finely chopped
    fresh flat-leaf parsley

Begin by cooking the bacon. Heat 1 teaspoon of the olive oil in a heavy-based frying pan and cook the bacon over a medium-low heat until just crisp. Cut into small pieces and set aside on a plate to cool.

Heat the remaining oil for the risotto in a heavy-based saucepan and fry the onion until it begins to soften. Add the rice and stir over a medium heat for 2–3 minutes. Add the wine and let it bubble up, stirring until absorbed. Gradually add the hot stock, a ladleful at a time, making sure that each ladleful has been absorbed before you add the next. Stir continuously until you have used up all the stock, by which time the rice should be soft. About 5 minutes before you think the rice is cooked, stir in the spinach. Finally, beat in the lemon zest, butter and seasoning. Keep warm and set aside.

Heat the pan you used for the bacon over a medium heat and cook the scallops for 2 minutes on each side until browned and opaque; be careful not to overcook them. Season and transfer to a plate. Deglaze the pan by pouring in the wine (or chicken stock) and letting it bubble up briefly.

To serve, pile the risotto onto a serving dish, lay the scallops on top, sprinkle over the bacon bits and drizzle over the deglazed juices from the scallop pan. Garnish with some chopped parsley.

Sirloin Steak Salad with Creamy Horseradish Dressing

My husband hates salad but loves steak, so this is my crafty way of getting him to eat a bit of the dreaded green stuff. I do actually do extra garlic bread – and sometimes an extra steak – for him to have on the side to keep him smiling. As for me, I pour a small glass of red wine to keep myself smiling.

Serves 2	9g FAT	2.4g SATURATES	6.8g SUGARS	1.37g SALT	315 CALORIES

1 x 200g lean sirloin steak
100g green beans
1 teaspoon olive oil
freshly ground black pepper
1 bag of mixed leaf salad
a handful of organic watercress
a handful of rocket
6 radishes, thinly sliced
8 cherry tomatoes

For the dressing
1 teaspoon creamed horseradish
2 tablespoons low-fat salad cream
2 teaspoons water
zest of 1 unwaxed lemon and
    1 tablespoon lemon juice
salt and freshly ground
    black pepper

For the herby garlic bread
4 thin slices of French bread
olive oil spray
1 garlic clove, peeled and
    crushed
sprinkling of dried mixed herbs

Take the steak out of the fridge half an hour before you want to eat. Steam the green beans until just tender; drain under cold running water and set aside. Mix together all the dressing ingredients in a small bowl and season with a little salt and plenty of black pepper.

Heat a griddle pan until nice and hot, rub both sides of the steak with the tiniest bit of oil and sprinkle with lots of black pepper. Put it on the griddle and cook for about a minute on each side if you want it to be rare. Transfer to a warm plate and set aside to rest for 2 minutes; this will ensure the steak stays tender and juicy.

To make the herby garlic bread, spray both sides of the French bread thinly with olive oil, sprinkle with the garlic and herbs and cook over a medium heat in the griddle pan you used for the steak.

Take a big platter and scatter it with the salad leaves, watercress, rocket, radish, green beans and cherry tomatoes. Thinly slice the steak, lay it on top of the salad and drizzle with the horseradish dressing. Accompany with the garlic bread.

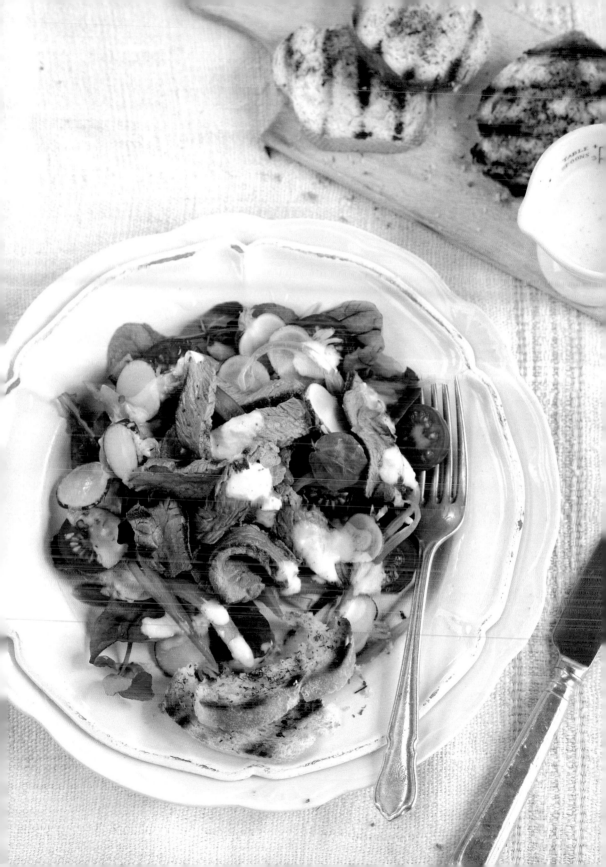

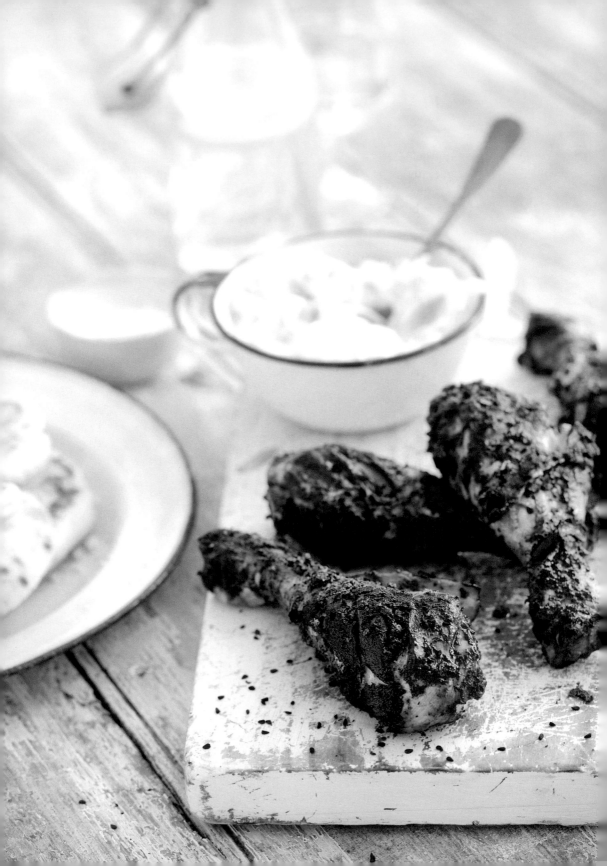

Tandoori Chicken with Tzatziki

Now don't judge me for putting red food colouring in this recipe for tandoori chicken. You see, I just can't help it – for me, it just doesn't feel right unless it is a lurid bright pink. Please feel free to leave it out, but I think you'll be missing out. This is best cooked on a barbecue, but you can always grill it.

Serves 2   8g FAT ┊ 3.6g SATURATES ┊ 8.6g SUGARS ┊ 1.12g SALT ┊ 362 CALORIES

2 small chicken breasts
2 small chicken drumsticks
juice of 1 lemon
2 teaspoons ground paprika
200ml low-fat Greek yogurt
1 tablespoon tandoori paste
2 teaspoons grated fresh
    root ginger
2 garlic cloves, peeled
    and crushed
½ teaspoon ground cumin
¼ teaspoon dried chilli flakes
a few drops of red food colouring
    (optional)

For the tzatziki
150ml low-fat Greek yogurt
½ teaspoon dried mint
1 tablespoon finely chopped
    fresh mint, plus a few leaves,
    to garnish
½ garlic clove, peeled and finely
    minced
½ cucumber, peeled and finely
    cubed

To serve
1 teaspoon nigella seeds
2 light naan breads

Take the skin off the chicken and slash the flesh a couple of times using a sharp knife. Place the chicken in a bowl with the lemon juice and paprika, give it a good mix to coat it all over and pop it in the fridge for 15 minutes.

To make the tandoori sauce, combine all the other ingredients in a bowl and give them a really good mix. Add the chicken and set aside in the fridge to marinate for at least 24 hours.

Remove the chicken from the fridge 30 minutes before you want to cook it and place it on a roasting rack to allow some of the sauce to drain off. Meanwhile, light the barbecue (or preheat the oven to 180°C/gas mark 4).

To make the tzatziki, put all the ingredients except the cucumber into a bowl and stir. Add the cucumber at the last minute.

Barbecue over white hot coals (or grill) for 5–6 minutes on each side, or until cooked through.

To serve, dry-fry the nigella seeds in a non-stick pan, sprinkle them over the cooked chicken and serve with the tzatziki and naan bread.

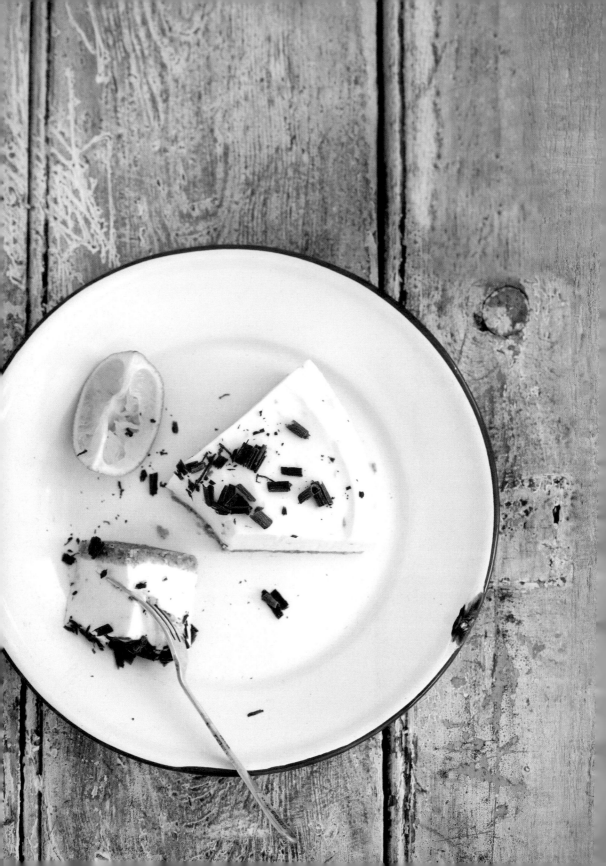

Decadent Desserts

'I firmly believe that everybody needs a little of what they fancy, or they end up having far too much of what they fancy!'

Decadent Desserts

I know what you're thinking. You're thinking, how on earth has she got away with putting so many naughty dessert recipes in a book with 'diet' in the title?! Is she bonkers?

Well firstly, I firmly believe everybody needs a little of what they fancy, or they end up having far too much of what they fancy! Honestly, whenever I've tried to completely cut out all things sweet I've eventually ended up bingeing on piles of the stuff instead of just enjoying the far more civilized single slice.

Basically, we can (almost) never have more than one helping of anything sweet if we want to be slim birds! There are a few things we can do to help us in this quest. Firstly, we must try not to make more than we need – and if there is anything left over, we need to immediately put it into the freezer, the bin or the dog! Better still, give it to your husband. Just ensure you do NOT leave it lying around, otherwise temptation will eventually get the better of you and you'll devour it in seconds, resulting in hours of self-loathing, which can usually only be soothed (momentarily) by... you guessed it, more sugar! How nuts are we?

Now, I hate rules. In fact, for most of my life I have acted like a complete idiot by routinely breaking most of the rules I've come across or that I've had foisted upon me. I say 'idiot' because most of those rules were usually in place for good reason!

As a child I was a nightmare, a classic madam. If there was a sign asking me to keep off the grass I couldn't wait to run across it. If homework was supposed to be in on a Monday, there was no way I was going to hand it in until at least Wednesday. And without too much effort at all I can conjure up the faces of at least five teachers from my dim and distant past who would all undoubtedly confirm (through gritted teeth) what a challenge I was!

I've been no better for most of my adult life, either. Why have a sensible glass or two of wine when I really want six? 'Go on, have six,' I would say. Why have one measly slice of cake when I really want three? 'Just have three,' I would say. Idiotic behaviour; behaviour that's helped me get really nice and fat! What a rebel I was... a greedy, fat rebel!

So when I decided I'd had enough of being the 'fat bird' and that I wanted to change, I knew there were going to have to be some (but not too many) rules put in place. If I wanted to feel slim, fit and healthy, if I wanted to buy clothes because I loved them rather than just because I could get into them, some kind of self-control was going to have to happen. Yes folks, it was a horrible shock but I knew that it was time to tell myself that I had to grow up a little, and finally accept that I simply couldn't have everything I wanted. I could no longer think and behave like a fat woman; I had to change my behaviour.

From now on I had to start behaving like... wait for it... the slim birds (a.k.a. the aliens). You know the ones I mean: the ones that only occasionally have a piece of cake and then eat it really slowly, casually – coolly, even – with a fork, while staying fully engaged in whatever else is going on around them. Crikey, the only way I knew how to eat dessert was with my head down, in the trough, practically inhaling it, oblivious to all else going on around me, only coming up for air, wild eyed and desperate for another slice!

Well, no more. My size 12 jeans feel so much better than that second helping ever tasted. And you'll notice how I only say 'second helping', there's absolutely no way I'm giving up the first one.

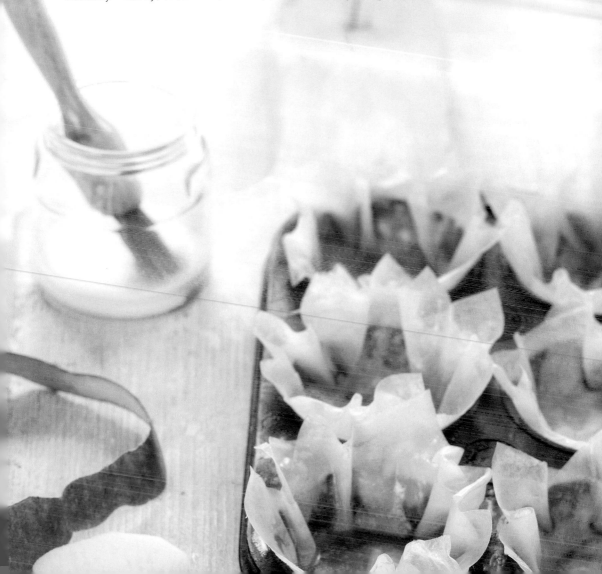

Puffy Fruit Bake

This is basically a sweet Yorkshire pudding with added cherries. It's a great choice for when you fancy a bit of sweet stodge – which, if you're anything like me, is all the time! If I happen to have some low-calorie cream in the fridge, I'll allow myself a drizzle of it over the top of my Puffy Bake – well, why not, it's only a drizzle!

Serves 6 | 3g FAT | 0.8g SATURATES | 49g SUGARS | 0.17g SALT | 279 CALORIES

85g plain flour

50g caster sugar

3 eggs, beaten

300ml skimmed milk

1 x 800g tin of pitted cherries, thoroughly drained (or whatever fruit you fancy)

icing sugar for dusting

Preheat the oven to 220°C/gas mark 7. Put the flour and sugar into a mixing bowl and make a well in the centre. Beat together the eggs and milk in a jug and gradually pour into the well, whisking the whole time until you have a smooth batter.

Arrange the cherries across the base of a 1.5 litre pudding dish and pour the batter on top. Bake for 25 minutes until puffed up and golden. Dust with icing sugar.

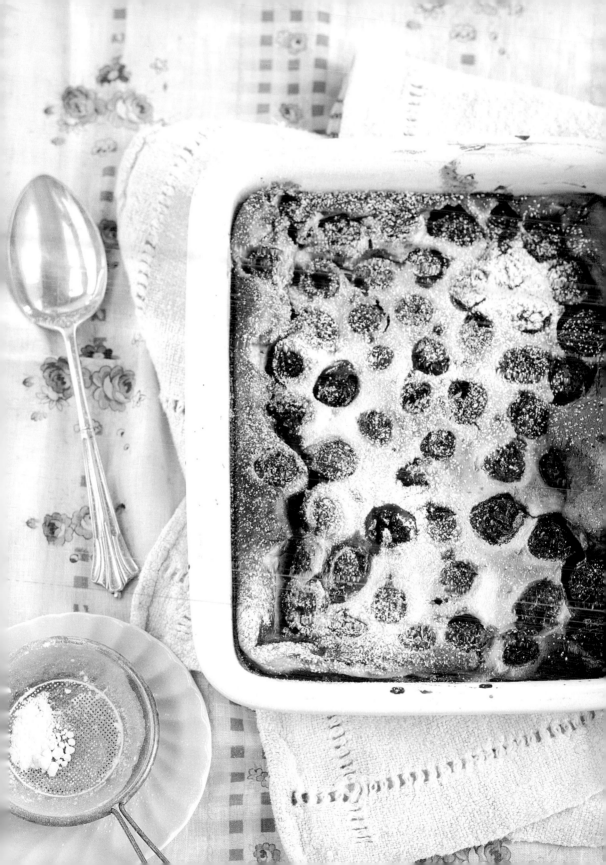

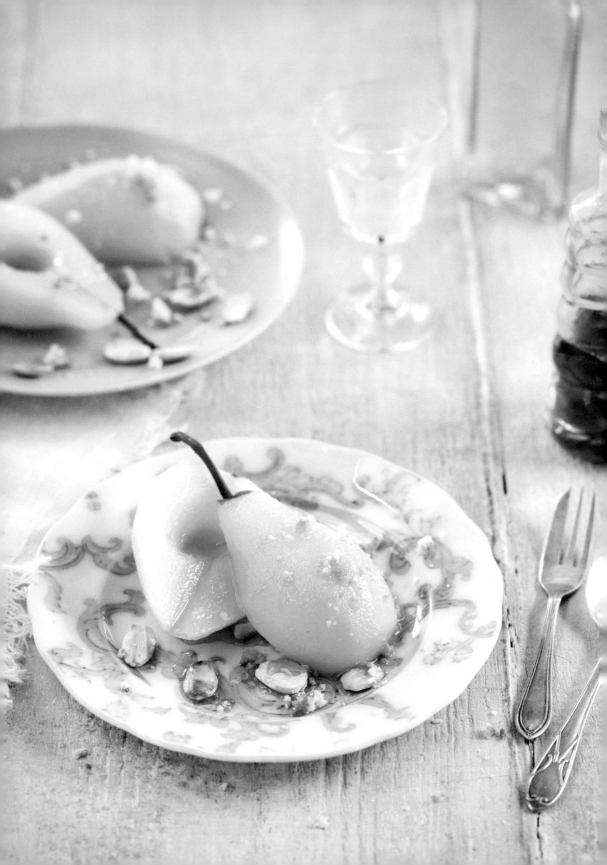

Cinnamon, Maple Syrup and Pear Crumble

This is a beautifully light dessert that is also incredibly easy to make. In fact, my nine-year-old can make it on her own from start to finish! So, the next time you have an urgent need for a treat, whip up this up. You won't be disappointed.

Serves 4   8g FAT | 0.9g SATURATES | 23.5g SUGARS | 0.11g SALT | 195 CALORIES

4 ripe pears, peeled, cored and halved
2 tablespoons best-quality maple syrup
4 amaretto biscuits, crumbled
50g roasted almonds
4 dessertspoons low-fat crème fraîche (or low-fat vanilla ice cream)

Place the pears in a pan, cover with water and poach very gently for 8–10 minutes (depending on their size) until tender, then drain.

Put the poached pears into a serving dish, drizzle with maple syrup and top with the crumbled amaretto biscuits and roasted almonds. Serve with crème fraîche (or low-cal ice cream).

Try to eat well without guilt. Your body is wonderful and deserves to be loved and nourished. Eating healthy foods with a positive attitude means you are far less likely to go scuttling off for a guilt-ridden biscuit tin binge!'

Coffee and Walnut Cake

I truly love cake, any kind of cake – chocolate cake, lemon drizzle cake, rock cakes, fairy cakes, apple cake and ginger cake. You name it, if it has cake after it, I will love it. In fact, as far as I'm concerned, any time of day is cake o'clock. But, of course, I can no longer indulge in cake in the same way as I used to in the past – otherwise, I'd be back up to a size 18 before I could say 'more cake please'. But neither am I going to give up cake completely. Oh no, life wouldn't be worth living without cake!

Serves 6 | 28g FAT | 4.7g SATURATES | 22.1g SUGARS | 1.03g SALT | 503 CALORIES

2 teaspoons instant espresso coffee granules

225g self-raising flour

1 teaspoon baking powder

50g ground almonds

80g caster sugar

25g chopped walnuts

2 eggs

250g low-fat Greek yogurt

75ml sunflower oil, plus extra for greasing

icing sugar, for dusting

8 walnut halves

For the filling

2 teaspoons instant espresso coffee granules

200g Philadelphia Extra Light cream cheese

1 tablespoon vanilla extract

2 tablespoons icing sugar

Preheat the oven to 180°C/gas mark 4. Lightly grease and line a 20cm round loose-based cake tin that is 6cm deep. To make the cake, combine the espresso coffee granules with 2 teaspoons warm water in a little cup. Sift the flour and baking powder into a large mixing bowl and stir in the almonds, caster sugar and chopped walnuts. Add the eggs, yogurt, oil and espresso coffee mixture and stir until everything is beautifully mixed.

Pour the batter into the prepared tin and bake for 40–45 minutes, or until a skewer inserted into the middle of the cake comes out clean. Leave to cool in the tin for 5 minutes, then turn out onto a wire rack to cool completely.

To make the filling, mix the espresso coffee granules with 2 teaspoons hot water and set aside. Using an electric whisk, whisk the cream cheese, vanilla extract and icing sugar in a bowl. Gradually pour in the coffee mixture and whisk again.

Slice the cake into two, fill with the filling and sandwich back together. To serve, sift icing sugar over the top and decorate with the walnut halves.

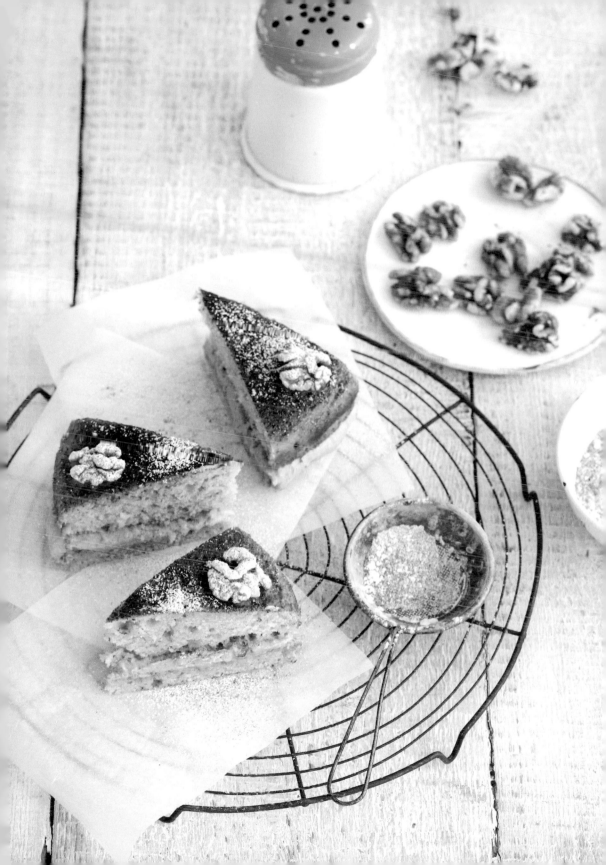

Banana Lollies

This is possibly the easiest dessert to make in the world – in fact, I just get the girls to do it while I have a lie down! Don't worry, only joking!

Makes 8 mini lollies

2g FAT | 0.2g SATURATES | 8.4g SUGARS | 0.06g SALT | 62 CALORIES

2 large bananas
200ml low-fat chocolate dessert
    or low-fat chocolate yogurt
2 tablespoons chopped
    hazelnuts, toasted and cooled
    if you have time
8 lolly sticks

Cut each banana into 4 pieces. Put a lolly stick into the cut end of each piece, dip into the chocolate dessert or yogurt, then roll in the toasted nuts.

Wrap each one individually in greaseproof paper and freeze for 3 hours.

'I am a great believer in keeping a food diary – and I don't mean in order to log boring calories! Write down what you have eaten and how you felt after eating it. Record when you have over-eaten and write down what else was going on in your life at the time. Were you sad? Lonely? Frightened? Did the doughnut really help?'

Chocolate Brownies

We all love to indulge in a chocolate brownie now and again but, my goodness, they are usually so fattening! Never fear, I am here to save the day with these little squares of loveliness. To set your mind at rest, I've replaced the butter with yogurt and used cocoa powder to get a deep chocolatey taste. Enjoy!

Makes 16 portions   3g FAT | 0.6g SATURATES | 11.5g SUGARS | 0.1g SALT | 94 CALORIES

85g self-raising flour
40g best-quality cocoa powder
160g golden caster sugar
125g natural set low-fat yogurt
2 eggs
1 teaspoon vanilla extract
25g chopped almonds

Preheat the oven to 180°C/gas mark 4. Line a 20cm square baking tray with baking paper.

Sift the flour and cocoa into a mixing bowl, then stir in the remaining ingredients, being careful not to overmix.

Spoon the mixture into the prepared tin and bake for about 25 minutes or until a skewer inserted into the centre comes out slightly gooey – which means that the brownies will still be nice and squidgy in the middle.

Set aside to cool in the tin before cutting into 16 squares – and only eat one! You can freeze them if you want, or they'll keep in an airtight container for a few days.

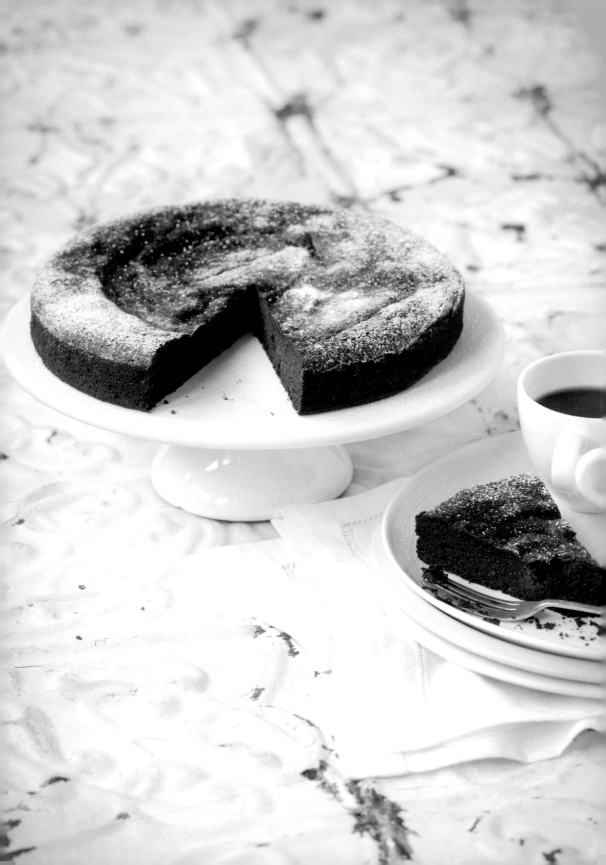

Auntie Jooooooolah's Cake

My little sister sees wheat as the devil incarnate, but she adores dark chocolate, so I always make this gorgeously moist cake for her when she comes to stay. My girls call it Auntie Jooooooolah's cake because, when they smell it cooking, they know she must be on her way!

P.S. My sisters' name is actually Julia but the girls couldn't say it when they were little, so it became Jooooooolah and stuck!

Serves 8	17g FAT	4.9g SATURATES	26.7g SUGARS	0.13g SALT	286 CALORIES

150g dark chocolate
35g cocoa powder
80ml water
100g ground almonds
100g soft brown sugar
4 eggs, separated
icing sugar for dusting

Preheat the oven to 180°C/gas mark 4. Line a 20cm round, loose-based cake tin that is 6cm deep with baking paper.

Place the chocolate in a heatproof bowl and set over a pan of gently simmering water, ensuring the water doesn't actually touch the bowl. Stir the chocolate until it melts.

Meanwhile, put the cocoa powder and water in a large mixing bowl and whisk until smooth. Add the melted chocolate, ground almonds, sugar and egg yolks and whisk well to combine.

In a separate bowl, whisk the egg whites until soft peaks form. Gently fold them into the cake mixture.

Pour the batter into the prepared tin and bake for 40–50 minutes or until a skewer inserted into the middle of the cake comes out clean. Remove the cake from the oven and set aside to cool in the tin for about half an hour, then turn out onto a wire rack to cool completely. Dust with icing sugar.

Lemon and Blueberry Sponges with Lemon Custard

What could be better on a wet Wednesday night after a miserable day at work – and having had a row with the fella – than this? Indeed, I find custard is probably one of the best things around for ironing out domestic ruffles and getting things back on course! Especially when poured over his head.

Serves 6   6g FAT | 1.3g SATURATES | 14.3g SUGARS | 0.52g SALT | 183 CALORIES

100g self-raising flour

½ teaspoon bicarbonate of soda

50g caster sugar

100ml skimmed milk

1 egg

zest of 1 unwaxed lemon

2 tablespoons light olive oil, plus extra for greasing

large handful of blueberries

For the custard

300g low-fat custard

zest and juice of ½ unwaxed lemon

Preheat the oven to 170°C/gas mark 3½ and brush 6 holes of a muffin tray with a tiny amount of oil.

Sift the flour into a large bowl, stir in the bicarbonate of soda and sugar and make a well in the centre. Beat together the milk, egg, lemon zest and oil in a jug. Pour the mixture into the well and give everything a quick stir with a wooden spoon; don't overmix it. Fold in the blueberries and divide the mixture between the prepared holes of the muffin tray. Bake for 15 minutes until the sponges are firm to the touch.

Pour the custard into a non-stick pan, add the lemon zest and juice and heat through. Pour over the lemon and blueberry sponges to serve.

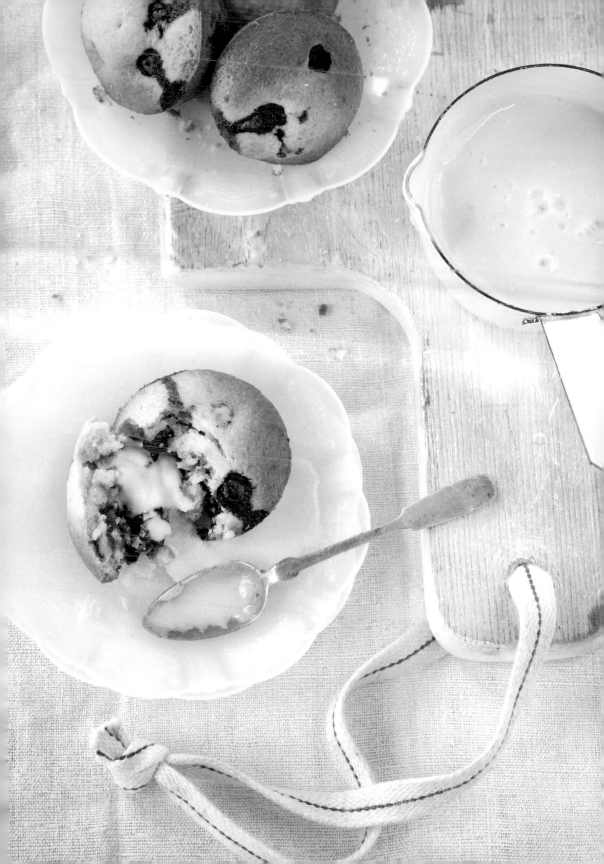

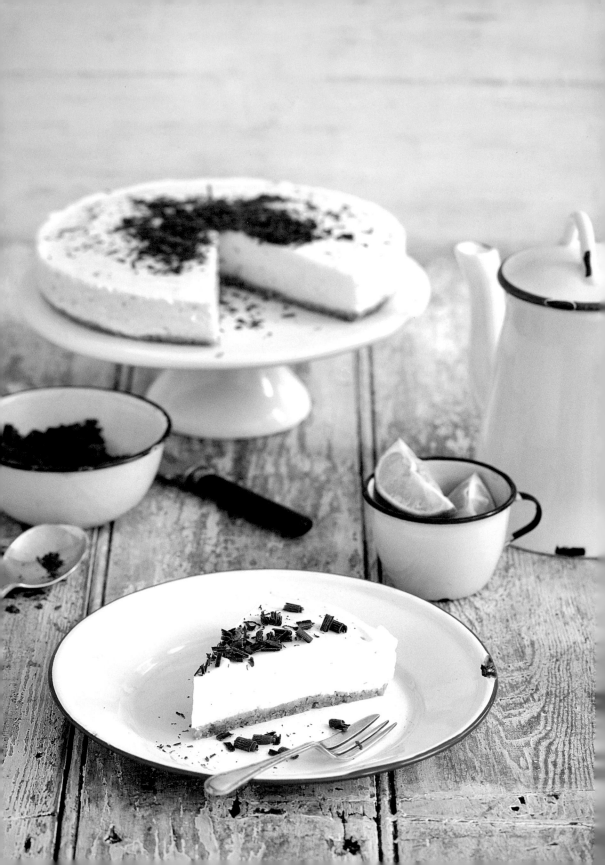

Lime and Chocolate Cheesecake

This is my daughter Maddies' favourite pudding. She just loves any kind of cheesecake, even a low-fat/sugar one – but, of course, she has no idea it's a low-fat/sugar one because it tastes gorgeous!

Serves 6	10g FAT	4.7g SATURATES	35g SUGARS	0.83g SALT	342 CALORIES

80g light digestive biscuits
50g light butter
4 sheets of gelatine
Zest of 2 and juice of 3
    unwaxed limes
200g Philadelphia Light
    cream cheese
500g Quark cheese
150g Splenda sugar
4 cubes of dark chocolate, grated

To make the base, put the digestive biscuits in a polythene bag and bash with a rolling pin until they become crumbs. Melt the butter in a non-stick saucepan and stir in the biscuit crumbs. Press into a 20cm springform cake tin and pop in the fridge to firm up for an hour.

Place the gelatine sheets in a saucepan, cover with cold water and set aside to soak according to packet instructions. Then squeeze in the lime juice and dissolve the gelatine over a low heat.

Whisk the cream cheese, Quark and sugar together in a bowl and stir in the lime zest. Pour in the gelatine mixture and beat well with a wooden spoon or electric whisk. Spoon onto the biscuit base and pop into the fridge for 3–4 hours until set. Sprinkle the grated chocolate over the top just before serving.

Sweet and Spicy Apple Pies

Mmmmm... pastry, brown sugar and cinnamon – ingredients that are just made for each other. I like to serve these little pies of loveliness warm with a small scoop of vanilla ice cream. The only problem is that I can't wait for them to cool down, so I end up eating them blisteringly hot, and burning my tongue!

Serves 4	4g FAT	0.9g SATURATES	17.5g SUGARS	0.25g SALT	142 CALORIES

2 dessert apples, peeled, cored and diced

1 teaspoon ground ginger, plus extra for sprinkling

1 teaspoon ground cinnamon, plus extra for sprinkling

2 heaped tablespoons raisins or sultanas

3 sheets of filo pastry

2 tablespoons light butter, melted

2 teaspoons soft dark brown sugar

low-fat custard, cream or ice cream, to serve

Preheat the oven to 180°C/gas mark 4. Have a non-stick muffin tin ready (you will only need 4 moulds).

Put the apples, spices and dried fruit into a pan with a couple of tablespoons water, bring up to the bubble and simmer until the apples are soft but still holding their shape. Pour the mixture into a sieve and set aside to drain.

Cut each sheet of filo pastry into 4 equal squares. Lay 4 of the squares on your worksurface and brush lightly with melted butter. Arrange 4 more squares on top, with their points offset, and brush again. Top with the remaining sheets of pastry, brush lightly again and press each stack into a muffin mould.

Fill the centre of each pastry case with some of the apple mixture, sprinkle the tops with brown sugar and dust with a little more cinnamon or ginger, or both, if you wish. Bake for 8–10 minutes. Serve with a little low-fat custard, cream or ice cream.

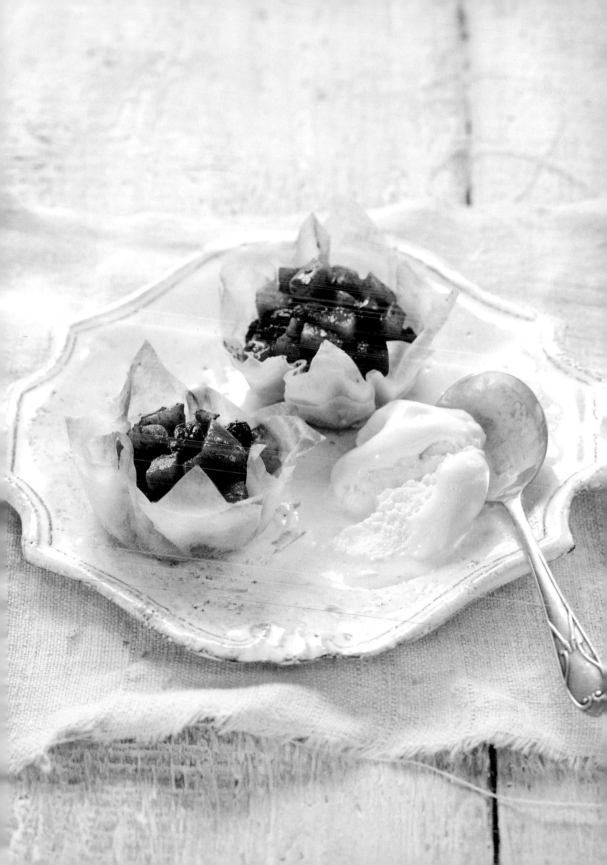

Pancakes with Raspberry Topping

You could swap the raspberries in this recipe for any berries you fancy. If you're serving them at a dinner party, but don't want to spend too much time away from your guests – I sometimes love to spend time away from my guests! – simply make everything beforehand and warm the pancakes through when you're ready.

Serves 4 | 2g FAT | 0.6g SATURATES | 11.9g SUGARS | 0.14g SALT | 187 CALORIES

For the pancakes
125g plain flour
1 medium egg
300ml skimmed milk
vegetable oil spray

For the raspberry topping
250g raspberries
2 tablespoons freshly squeezed
    orange juice
1–2 tablespoons caster sugar
1 teaspoon vanilla extract

To serve
1 teaspoon icing sugar stirred
    into 4 tablespoons half-fat
    crème fraîche

To make the pancake batter, blend or whisk together the flour, egg and milk. Set aside to rest while you make the raspberry topping.

Put the raspberries, juice, sugar and vanilla extract into a saucepan and heat very gently until the raspberries begin to bubble slightly and soften. Take off the heat and set aside.

To cook the pancakes, heat a small non-stick frying pan over a medium heat and spray with vegetable oil. Pour a little batter into the pan, swirl it around and cook gently until it begins to bubble on the top. Flip over and fry on the other side. The whole process should take about 2–3 minutes and the mixture should yield 8 pancakes. You can spray the pan before cooking each pancake, if you think it's necessary.

When all the pancakes are cooked, put 2, folded over, onto each plate. Spoon the raspberries over the top and accompany with a tablespoon of the sweetened crème fraîche.

Raspberry and Rosewater Jelly

As a kid, I used to love the moment at birthday parties when the jelly and ice cream would come out, especially if it was super-tacky, lurid-coloured jelly with budget ice cream – oh well, we all have to grow up at some point!

Serves 6	trace FAT	0.0g SATURATES	10.0g SUGARS	0.04g SALT	56 CALORIES

55g caster sugar
50ml rosewater
4 leaves of gelatine
150g raspberries
raspberry ice cream, to serve

'Enjoy a little of what you fancy, but not too much! My size 12 jeans feel so much better than that second helping ever tasted.'

Combine the sugar with 400ml water in a pan and stir over a low heat until the sugar has dissolved. Bring up to the boil, then reduce heat and simmer for 5 minutes. Take the pan off the heat.

Combine the rosewater with 350ml water in a large bowl. Add the gelatine leaves and set aside to soak for about 5 minutes until the gelatine has softened. Take the gelatine out of the water, squeeze out as much liquid as possible, holding it over the rosewater to catch the drips, and put it into the pan with the hot sugar syrup. Whisk vigorously until the gelatine has completely dissolved, then pour the syrup into the bowl with the rosewater, whisking really well.

Divide the mixture between 6 individual glasses and pop in the fridge to set for about an hour. Once the jelly has set slightly, add the raspberries. Put back in the fridge for at least 4 hours until completely set. Serve with a smug smile and a spoonful of raspberry ice cream.

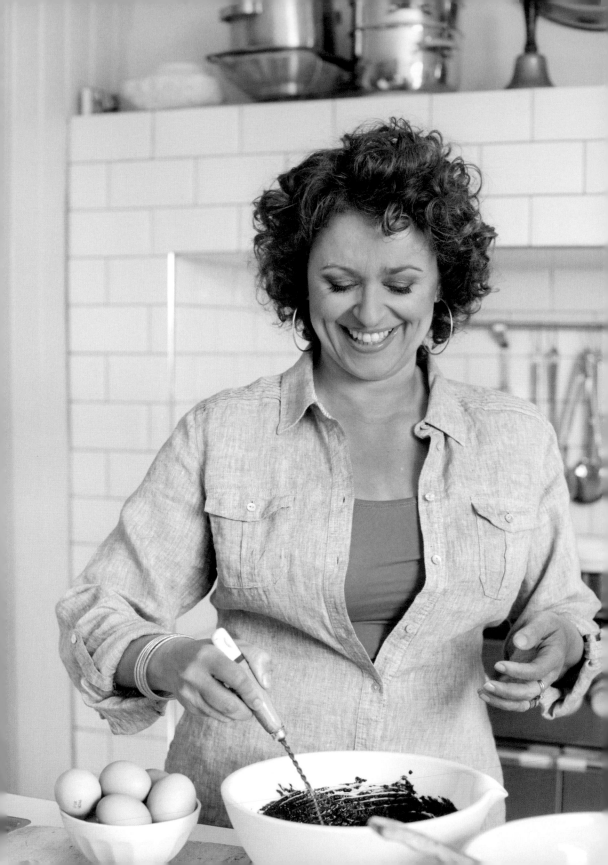

Chocolate Meringues

Meringues are a great dessert because they don't have any fat whatsoever, but they feel so naughty. I make these when I have my girlfriends over for dinner as meringues don't seem to bring the same cheer to men as they do to women – weird, huh?

Makes 6 meringues

2g FAT | 0.2g SATURATES | 17.7g SUGARS | 0.25g SALT | 93 CALORIES

4 large egg whites
¼ teaspoon cream of tartar
100g caster sugar
2 teaspoons cocoa powder

To decorate
1 tablespoon chopped hazelnuts
1 teaspoon cocoa powder

Preheat the oven to 150°C/gas mark 2. Line a baking tray with baking paper.

In a large clean bowl, beat the egg whites with an electric mixer set to a slow to medium speed until they are foamy, then add the cream of tartar and continue to whisk until your whites form soft peaks.

Add the sugar, a tablespoon at a time, and continue whisking at a higher speed until stiff peaks form.

Sift in the cocoa powder and gently fold in with a metal spoon – don't mix it in completely, though, as we are after swirls of chocolate.

Spoon the mixture onto your prepared baking sheet so you end up with 6 meringues altogether. Sprinkle them evenly with hazelnuts, dust lightly with cocoa powder and bake for 1 hour.

Raspberry and Chocolate Mousse Pots

My mum is always watching her weight, so I created these little pots for her because they are lovely and light and include two of her very favourite things – raspberries and chocolate. Yum!

Serves 4	14g FAT	6.1g SATURATES	20.1g SUGARS	0.05g SALT	222 CALORIES

75g dark chocolate
2 large organic egg whites
1 tablespoon caster sugar
4 tablespoons reduced-fat crème fraîche
350g raspberries

Break up the chocolate into a heatproof bowl set over a pan of barely simmering water, ensuring the water doesn't touch the bowl. Stir the chocolate until it melts. Once it has melted, set aside to cool.

Meanwhile, using an electric whisk, whisk the egg whites until stiff. Slowly add the sugar and whisk again until stiff.

Place the crème fraîche in a bowl and stir in the cooled chocolate. Gently fold in the egg white mixture. Divide the raspberries between 4 individual pots and top with the chocolate mousse. Pop into the fridge for 4 hours to set.

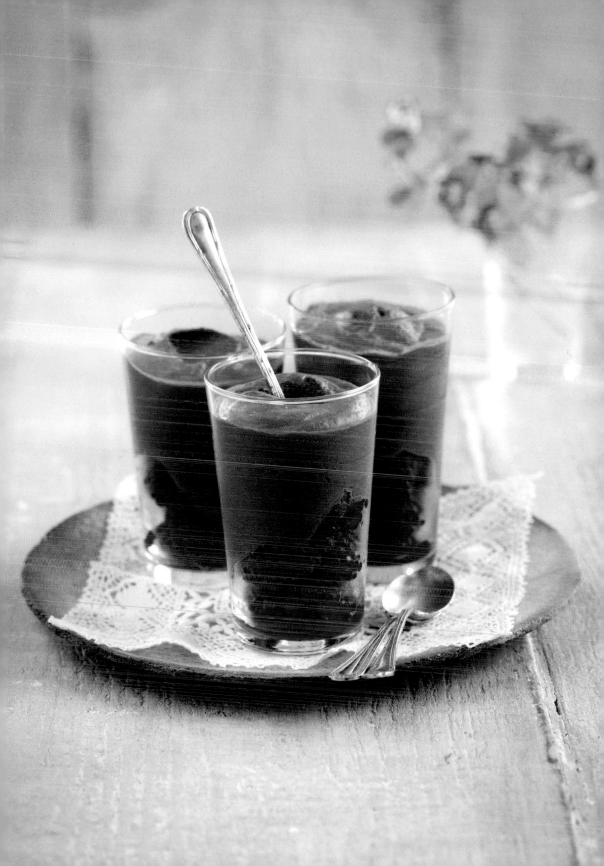

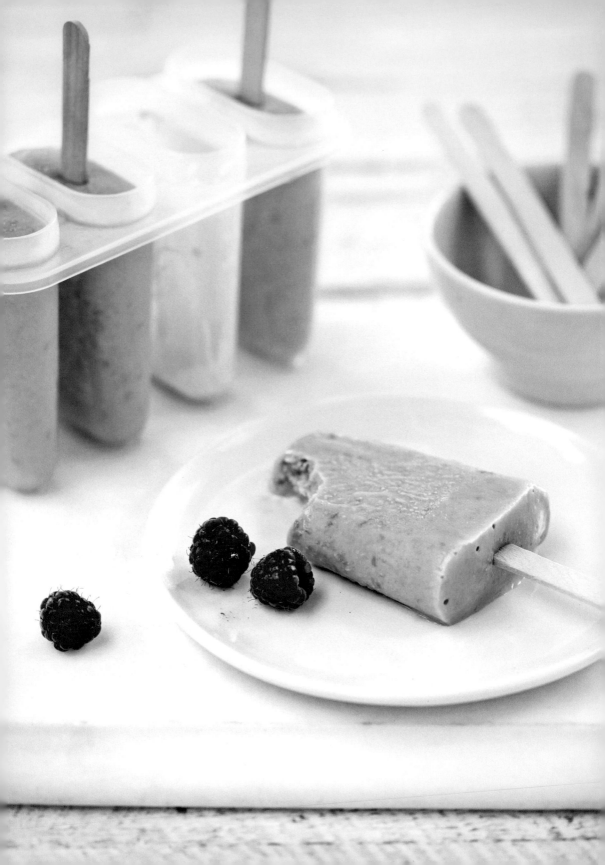

Raspberry and Almond Ice Pops

Ice cream, ice cream, we all scream for ice cream! These delicious ice-creamy pops will keep the whole family happy on a hot day – and on a cold one too, come to think of it.

Makes 12

0.4g FAT | 0.1g SATURATES | 22.6g SUGARS | 0.12g SALT | 101 CALORIES

400g ripe raspberries
200ml almond milk
1 x 400g can light
   condensed milk
1 teaspoon vanilla extract

Put all the ingredients into a food processor and blitz. Pour into 12 ice lolly moulds and freeze.

'So many of us munch out of boredom rather than hunger – so next time you catch yourself heading to the fridge simply because you're bored, ask yourself whether you're really hungry. If you're not, try and find another way to relieve your boredom!

Banoffee Dessert

Anything with banoffee in the title seems to whip people into a frenzy! Hardly surprising, though, since it is usually packed full of fat, sugar and a vast amount of calories. You might not expect to find banoffee in a diet book but, as I always say, where there's a will, there's a way!

Serves 4 | 6g FAT | 1.5g SATURATES | 29.9g SUGARS | 0.4g SALT | 213 CALORIES

4 light digestive biscuits

4 scoops of low-fat vanilla ice cream

4 tablespoons caramel sauce

2 bananas, sliced

1 teaspoon vanilla extract

a squeeze of lemon juice

1 teaspoon grated dark chocolate or cocoa powder

Break up the biscuits and divide equally between 4 glasses. Top with the ice cream, caramel sauce and sliced banana. Add a few drops of vanilla and a squeeze of lemon juice to each and sprinkle over the grated chocolate.

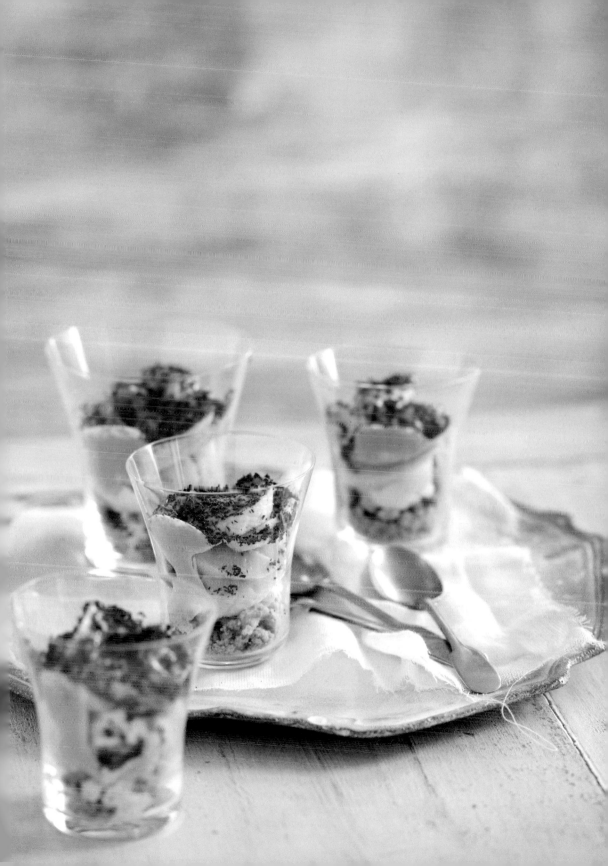

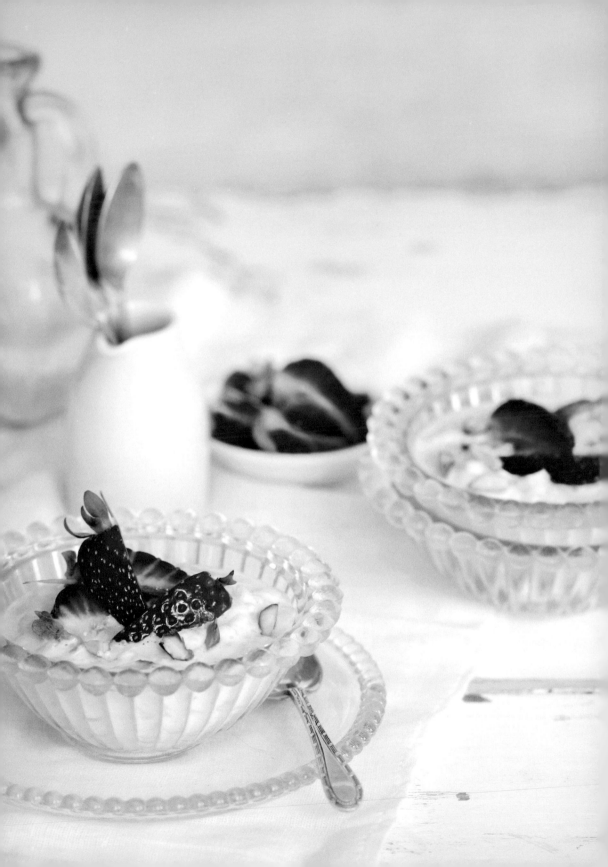

Middle Eastern-Style Rice Pudding with Rosewater and Strawberries

I'm going to be honest, I'm not a mad fan of rice pudding – but the rest of the family most certainly are, and they particularly love this Middle East-inspired one I've created. But even though I don't like eating this dish, I certainly love making it!

Serves 4   5g FAT | 1.7g SATURATES | 17.7g SUGARS | 0.2g SALT | 297 CALORIES

600ml skimmed milk
1 teaspoon vanilla extract
200g pudding rice
2 tablespoons sugar
4 tablespoons reduced-fat cream
1 tablespoon rosewater
100g chopped strawberries
a small handful of pistachio nuts

Pour the milk and vanilla extract into a microwavable mixing bowl and stir in the rice and sugar. Cover with clingfilm and pierce with a fork. Cook in the microwave on a high setting for 5 minutes, then give it a stir, wait for a minute and cook for a further 5 minutes. Check that all the milk has soaked into the rice; if it hasn't, pop it back in the microwave for an extra minute.

To serve, stir in the cream and rosewater and top with the strawberries and pistachio nuts.

Exotic Baked Figs

This is a gorgeously exotic, fragrant dessert that should be made illegal because it's so easy to rustle up. But – and it's a big but – do not bother to make it unless you can get really good figs.

Serves 4 | 6g FAT | 0.9g SATURATES | 23.8g SUGARS | 0.04g SALT | 176 CALORIES

4 tablespoons agave syrup

3 tablespoons brandy

8 ripe figs

4 teaspoons rosewater

4 tablespoons pistachio nuts

4 tablespoons low-fat Greek
   yogurt

Preheat the grill to moderate. Pour the agave syrup and brandy into a little jug.

Make a deep cross in the top of each fig and then open it out a bit. They will look absolutely beautiful, so don't be tempted to swipe one straight away!

Put the figs into a roasting tin and drizzle over the agave syrup and brandy mixture. Pop under the grill and cook for 6–8 minutes until they are nicely softened – but keep your eye on them as you don't want them to burn.

Shower the figs with a little rosewater, then sprinkle the nuts on top. Serve warm with the Greek yogurt.

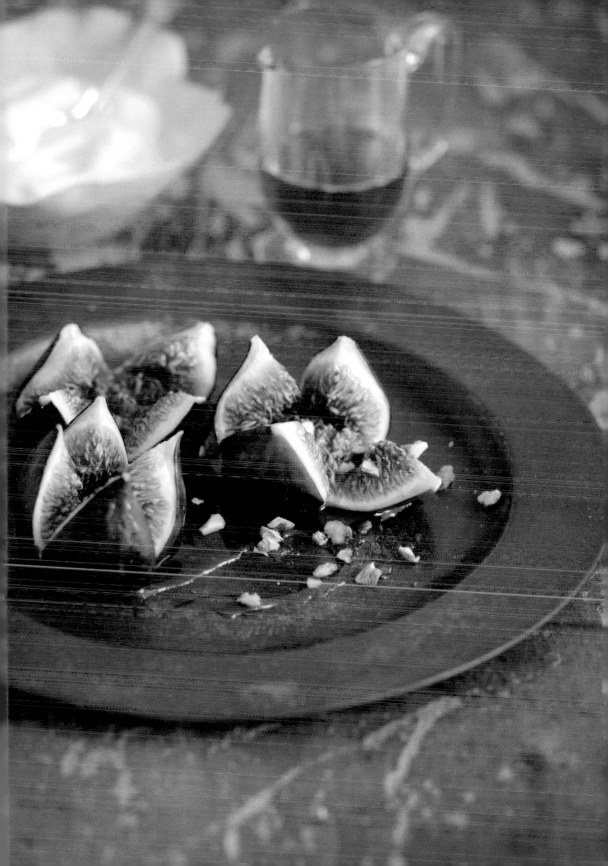

Index

Acknowledgements

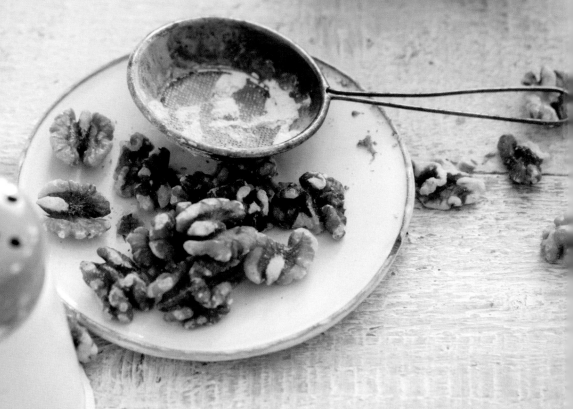

A huge thank you to Polly Webb-Wilson, Keiko Oikawa and Iris Bromet for creating a book that *looks* so beautiful, and by dint of that making *me* look so classy!

Thank you to my editor Judith Hannam for all her hard work, and for letting me keep half the exclamation marks I actually used!!!!

Thank you to my agent Neil Howarth at Urban for all the graft (nod, nod, wink, wink!) that you put in to make this book happen!

Thank you so much, Mum. I literally couldn't have written this book without you. x